Current Therapy of Communication Disorders

GENERAL PRINCIPLES OF THERAPY

Upcoming volumes in the series:

Language Handicaps in Children

Language Handicaps in Adults

Phonologic-Articulatory Disorders

Voice Disorders

Stuttering Disorders

Dysarthria and Apraxia

Hearing Disorders

Current Therapy of Communication Disorders

GENERAL PRINCIPLES OF THERAPY

edited by
William H. Perkins, Ph.D.
University of Southern California

1982
Thieme-Stratton Inc.
New York

Georg Thieme Verlag
Stuttgart • New York

Acknowledgment
I am grateful to Janis Costello and Richard Curlee for their guidance in the selection of therapies and authors for this volume.

Publisher: Thieme-Stratton Inc.
381 Park Avenue South
New York, New York

Cover typography by M. Losaw

Printed in the United States of America

CURRENT THERAPY OF COMMUNICATION DISORDERS

General Principles of Therapy
edited by William H. Perkins

TSI ISBN 0–86577–077–8

GTV ISBN 3–13–636701–4

Library of Congress catalog card number 82–51143.

Last digit is print number 5 4 3 2 1

Contents

Contributing Authors

Janis M. Costello, Ph.D.
University of California, Santa Barbara

Lois W. Douglass, M.A.
Private practice, Pasadena, California

Raymond D. Kent, Ph.D.
University of Wisconsin, Madison

Deborah R. Klevans, Ph.D.
Private practice, State College, Pennsylvania

John T. Lybolt, Ph.D.
Boys Town Institute for Communication Disorders in Children, Omaha, Nebraska

Clyde L. Rousey, Ph.D.
Private practice, Topeka, Kansas

Gerald M. Siegel, Ph.D.
University of Minnesota, Minneapolis

C. Woodruff Starkweather, Ph.D.
Temple University, Philadelphia, Pennsylvania

PREFACE

Roughly a billion dollars is invested annually in the clinical service of speech, language, and hearing disorders. Were this service provided to only one person, our best effort would be mandatory. The magnitude of the investment merely heightens the importance of our clinical responsibility.

This text is the first volume of a larger effort to help meet this responsibility. All eighty-seven chapters in the series are intended for the practicing clinician, who needs a convenient reference for therapy of any problem of speech, language, or hearing. The series contains as many chapters as are required to present all the forms of therapy that should be differentiated for disorders of language, articulation, voice, fluency, and hearing in children and adults. One could call this a "distinctive feature approach" in the sense that therapy of any disorder that is distinguished from therapy of another disorder by at least one feature of treatment warrants a separate chapter.

To avoid repetition, general procedures for learning new responses, transferring them to daily life, and making them permanent, are presented in this first volume. Each general technique is described from the standpoint of whatever theory of learning it is mainly derived. For example, response shaping is presented as an operant procedure, modeling as a procedure of cognitive learning theory. Thus, the following approaches to therapy in the left hand column are described in terms of the appropriate theory or principles in the right hand column.

Procedures	Theory or Principle of Learning
Acquisition of language and cognitive skills	Cognitive learning theory
Acquisition of motor speech skills	Counseling
Response shaping	Classical conditioning
Imitation	Motor learning theory
Modeling	Operant theory
Automatization	Psychotherapy
Reinforcement and punishment	
Counter conditioning	
Transfer	
Generalization	
Maintenance	
Self-Management	
Attitude adjustment of client's family	
Personality adjustment	

These procedures are purposely not repeated in the specific disorders chapters so that the focus can be maintained on the steps used to adapt treatment to the specific problem. The intent is for this volume to provide a review of general procedures that are derived from a larger theoretical framework. In this manner, each chapter of all the volumes is a free standing, terse, complete procedural account of a specific therapy as practiced by the author for a specific type of disorder.

The focus of this volume, as well as the others, is exclusively on treatment. Matters of assessment, diagnosis, and rationale are included only to the extent that they are needed to clarify characteristics of the person for whom the therapy is intended, and the reasons for it. Credibility of the therapy is embedded in credibility of the authors, who were selected on the best advice I could obtain. Asking them to describe what they do was tantamount to asking them to evaluate our treatment-research literature. Because they must make the most responsible judgment they can for each person they serve, their treatment recognizes the research that has therapy-value and goes beyond science to include the intangible verities of clinical practice as an art.

William H. Perkins

GENERAL PRINCIPLES OF THERAPY

CHAPTER ONE

TECHNIQUES OF THERAPY BASED ON OPERANT CONDITIONING

Method of Janis M. Costello

PINPOINTING TARGET BEHAVIORS

The major hallmark of an operant conditioning approach is its reliance upon observable behavior. Assessment and treatment are hinged on the clinician's ability to pinpoint relevant behaviors that are appropriate for the learner. As long as selected target behaviors are readily observable (preferably by more than one person) and are quantifiable in terms of frequency and/or duration, they will probably be amenable to treatment through the principles of operant conditioning. It is the responsibility of the clinician to generate operational definitions of behaviors and processes that are appropriate for each client to acquire or change. In my own clinical work I use a combination of formal test measures, direct observations of the client's communicative behaviors in a variety of natural communication situations, and developmental data as a basis for formulating the target behaviors I pinpoint for treatment. In many cases I also ask the client, the client's family and teachers, and lay persons who observe videotapes of the client's communicative interactions to tell me what they think needs changing in a client's behavior to make it more normal.

I combine all of these sources of information to select one or more target behaviors for treatment. In some cases I may select a behavior that is already in the client's repertoire, but which I intend to increase in its frequency of occurrence, such as question-asking in an emotionally disturbed child with inadequate social communicative skills. For other clients I may concentrate on reduction or elimination of a particular form of behavior from their talking repertoire, such as elimination of moments of stuttering. For still other clients the desired behavior may not exist in their repertoire, and so it has to be built in through shaping and successive approximation techniques. An example of this might be the conceptualization of time dimensions demonstrated by the appropriate use of past tense markers in a client's expressive language. It is not at all unusual, of course, to find clients for whom the treatment I design contains a combination of increasing, decreasing, and instating behaviors.

SELECTING FUNCTIONAL CONSEQUENCES

The basic premise of learning from an operant conditioning view is that behavior is controlled by its consequences. Therefore, a mandatory step in the planning of therapy is to determine or establish functional consequences to be used during the course of treatment. In general, I try to find stimuli that are convenient, quick to dispense, and, of course, functional for the client in question. For many clients I begin by establishing a token reinforcement system.

The most important components of a token system are the backup reinforcers that the client will exchange periodically for the tokens that have been earned. The power of the token reinforcement system rests with the selection of these backup reinforcers because it is the pairing of these reinforcers with the tokens that transforms the otherwise neutral tokens into conditioned positive reinforcers and enables them to maintain and increase correct responding during the treatment.

I select the backup reinforcers by first making a list of items that would seem to be potential reinforcers for a given client: those to which I have access, and those that could be provided by the parents or the client himself. Since this list must be geared to the particular individual, I spend some time during the pretreatment assessment sessions inquiring about favorite activities, hobbies, and the like. At this time I also explain about the opportunity to earn special items and certain privileges as speech improves during our sessions together. I share the list of potential positive reinforcers that I have made up with the client and ask him to suggest others that he would like to add to the list. When appropriate, I do the same thing with the parent or spouse. Then, depending on the age, I ask the client or the parent to rank each item on the "reinforcement menu" in terms of its judged value to the client. Then I pick the most highly rated items to use as backup reinforcers in the token reinforcement system. One of the advantages of such a system is that it provides a variety of reinforcers which help to maintain interest in the reinforcers available. As a general rule, I try to avoid selection of backup reinforcers that require a lot of time to administer (e.g., playing a game of backgammon) or are not immediately available at the time they are earned (e.g., watching a particular television program or having Mom stop for an ice cream cone on the way home), or those that are of rather high value and so should "cost" a great number of tokens (e.g., a new record album or one's weekly allowance). These are not good selections as backup reinforcers during the initial establishment and use of the token system because they either use up too much of the treatment time or they interject too much time between occurrence of the response and its token presentation and pairing of the backup reinforcer with the tokens. Later in the treatment sequence such delayed reinforcement becomes more appropriate.

I begin establishment of the token system as soon as seemingly appropriate backup reinforcers have been selected. I try to develop the token system during my assessment and evaluation sessions so that it is in place when treatment begins. In my clinic we use beans as tokens because they are handy, they make a nice, obvious sound when being dropped into a plastic cup, and they are inexpensive. Any arbitrarily selected stimulus can be used as a token, however, such as marking off squares on a prepared piece of paper, poker chips, beads, and so on.

I begin the first token training session by presenting to the client a choice of backup reinforcers and asking him to select the one he would like to work for first. After the item is selected, it (or a card designating what it is to be) is placed on the table near the client. Then I put 10 beans out on the table and explain briefly that when all 10 tokens are earned they may be exchanged for the selected item, activity, or privilege. Then we proceed to the activities planned for that session, and I present tokens frequently for various responses that are already in the client's repertoire such as looking at me when an instruction is presented, turning pages in the test booklet, sitting up straight, and the like. Essentially, then, the beans are "free," since no particular new response is required of the client. Each presentation of a token is also paired with my verbal praise so that my approval will also become a conditioned reinforcer for the client. When all 10 tokens have been presented, I stop the ongoing activity, ask the client to give me the beans earned, and in exchange give him the previously selected item. If it is a child with a toy, he is allowed to play with it momentarily and then he puts it away to take home with him (or the play activity is removed after a certain period of time). Then the batch of backup reinforcers is presented again and the client picks out the next thing he would like to work for. This time 20 tokens are on the table for him to earn. (I usually do not announce that more tokens are being added; I just do it.) This process continues for three or four sessions until the client has gradually learned that he has to fill an entire cup with tokens before he has earned the backup reinforcer and that he will not always fill a cup at each session. (He begins with the partially filled cup at the next session.)

At this point I am hoping that the tokens have become functional conditioned positive reinforcers, but I like to try to check this out to be sure. One way of doing that is to test the tokens on some neutral behavior before applying them to the treatment target behavior. I sometimes ask the client, for example, to name words at random, and I keep track of the parts of speech produced and then begin presenting praise and tokens for a particular part of speech, such as verbs, that had occurred at a somewhat low rate during the beginning of the task. Then I keep track to see if verbs increase in their frequency of occurrence. If they do, and if they return to a lower rate when I discontinue reinforcing them or reinforce another part of speech, then I have an idea that the tokens have become functional reinforcers, and I am (almost) ready to begin treatment.

Based on clinical experience and some laboratory data of my own and of others, it seems that the effectiveness of treatment is enhanced when feedback is provided both for correct and for incorrect responses. Therefore, after functional positive reinforcers have been selected, I also select stimuli to use as punishers. Typically, when a token reinforcement system is used, a simple and very effective punisher is response cost—the removal of a token immediately following an incorrect response. Usually I accompany this by saying "no" as well. Once again, testing these procedures on actual behavior is a better way of discovering if they are functional consequences than making those assumptions a priori or trying to judge this by the client's reactions. Punishing stimuli are simply ones that produce a reduction in the frequency of the behavior they follow. Especially when used in combination with positive reinforcers for appropriate behavior (which should always be the case), they do not need to be "mean" or intensely aversive stimuli. They simply act as stimuli the client would like to avoid and also provide added information so that the client can more quickly learn that some responses are acceptable (those that produce positive reinforcers) and some are not (those that produce removal of positive reinforcers or presentation of mildly aversive feedback).

It should be noted that reinforcing and punishing stimuli are not for children alone. Although the nature of the stimuli selected may be different, adult clients require and respond to contingencies in the same manner as children, and the selection of individualized, functional consequences is a mandatory step in the planning of their treatment as well.

DESIGNING TREATMENT PROGRAMS

Once I have determined appropriate target behaviors and effective positive and negative consequences, I am ready to plan the treatment program for a client. Programmed instruction combines the various principles of operant learning into a cohesive and systematic treatment approach. These principles are outlined only briefly here, since I have described them in detail elsewhere (see Selected References). Programmed instruction allows the client to learn complex behavior by beginning with simpler, smaller bits of behavior that are related to the selected target behavior and are already in the client's repertoire. By moving in small steps, as the treatment progresses, behavior becomes more complex, more independent, and more integrally stabilized into the client's repertoire. Further, learning is pleasant for the client because he is progressing toward his goal in a recognizable manner; he is earning lots of positive reinforcement along the way; he is learning without great struggle because he is mastering each level before moving to the next, and he is moving at a pace that is determined by his own speed of learning.

When I am working with clients, I tend not to rely on predesigned, commercially available treatment programs, although many of these are excellent. It is my feeling, however, that although there are many commonalities among clients with similar communicative disorders, no one program fits every client. Such a universal program would need to contain so many steps and provisions for the vagaries of some clients' behaviors that it would contain many steps not needed by a given client and still probably omit some required by another client. It is better, I feel, for clinicians to have the skill to design systematic and effective treatment programs for individual clients. Although many clients may follow essentially the same treatment plan, some of them start at different places in the sequence; some are able to skip steps that others have required; and some need intervening steps that no other client has ever needed. Furthermore, clinicians' selection of a target behavior for a given client should not be influenced by the convenience of already available treatment programs.

Programmed instruction is written so that for each small, progressive step of the teaching sequence, all of the information needed to conduct the teaching is specified. The program protocol describes, then, the particular response required of the client, the stimuli that will evoke that response, the positive and negative consequences that will follow correct and incorrect responses and how often these should be presented, how well the client must perform before moving on to the next step in the sequence, and how poorly he must perform before the program is adjusted to offset his failure. Changes occur in each of these program dimensions as the client advances through the program.

For example, as the program progresses, the responses required of the client become gradually more complex, more natural, and more like those appropriate to the natural environment. The stimuli presented to evoke treatment responses concurrently change so that the amount of help I am giving the client in terms of instructions, models to imitate, and particular stimuli to respond to diminishes, and evoking stimuli become more like the stimuli in the natural environment to which the client will eventually be responding. I also change the nature and frequency of positive reinforcement as the treatment sequence progresses. At the beginning of treatment, powerful but rather artificial reinforcers are used and are presented essentially for every correct response produced by the client. Likewise, every incorrect response is also given feedback. As the program moves away from this laboratory-like control to more natural uses of the targeted communicative behavior, the tokens (or whatever artificial reinforcers have been contingently arranged up to this point) are gently eased out and reinforcers that are primarily social, and likely to be found in the client's natural communicative environment, are used exclusively. Further, the reinforcement schedule slowly and subtly changes from the immediate and continuous reinforcement already described, to intermittent and delayed reinforcement schedules where only a few of the client's correct responses produce arranged reinforcement, and where that reinforcement may not be delivered immediately when the response occurs.

One further dimension of change that I make during the course of treatment is to add activities and contingencies that will promote eventual generalization and maintenance of treatment effects. Programming for generalization occurs throughout the acquisition phase of my treatment program and is generally the sole concern of the last phase of treatment plans. Some of the procedures I often incorporate into treatment for this purpose (beyond those of changing stimulus and reinforcement control already described) might be teaching the client to self-monitor and to provide his own positive and negative consequences for correct and incorrect responses, conducting the teaching concurrently in more than one environment and utilizing parents and peers as treatment agents, establishing rigorous pass criteria for critical steps of the treatment program to promote automatization of the newly acquired behavior, and moving the treatment setting into the natural environment.

MEASURING TREATMENT EFFECTIVENESS

The kind of individualized and efficient treatment described here is inherent in the principles of programmed instruction because sensitive measurement of treatment progress is an essential ingredient of programming. It is not possible for me to determine when a client has mastered a particular set of behaviors unless I am collecting data during treatment and I see that he can now produce a particular response, say, ten times in a row correctly. If that is what I have specified as an adequate level of performance, then I know that I can move on to the next step and that the client will be more likely to acquire that new behavior because he has mastered the previous one. On the other hand, I would be remiss as a teacher if I let my client struggle along in the treatment program without making substantial progress, because arranging and guaranteeing appropriate learning is my responsibility as the clinician. I need objective information about the client's learning before I determine that it is appropriate to move on or before I determine that I have made a programming error and need to devise a branch step because the client has gotten stuck somewhere along the way. And I need objective information before I can accurately decide that my client has successfully completed my treatment program and can be dismissed.

The fact that I am dealing with clearly observable and well-defined behavior at each step in my treatment plan allows me to collect precise data on the progress of the client so that I can make these move-ahead, fall-back, and dismissal decisions objectively. I generally calculate the number of trials required to meet the pass criterion and the percentage of correct responses for each step of a program. These data then tell me how the client is progressing and also give me information about the quality of my treatment program. When I see that a client is performing consistently above the 85 to 90 percent correct level on each step of the program, I know that he is doing well and that, therefore, I have done well. (Clinicians need reinforcement, too.) However, when I see that the client has failed a step (a fail criterion might be the occurrence of five consecutive incorrect responses), then I know that I have made a programming error for this client and that this step of the program needs revising or simplifying in some way. My treatment can be immediately responsive to the client's performance because the data tell me, response by response, how we are getting along.

Keeping response-by-response data during treatment also allows a clinician to become an experimenter. For example, while working with a particular client, one might wonder if using actual objects as stimuli rather than pictures might evoke more appropriate responses. If the clinician arranges the task so that for 20 consecutive trials objects are used, then for the next 20 trials pictures are presented, and these two conditions continue to be alternated a few times within the session, she can then calculate the percentage of correct responses evoked by each condition separately and judge whether there was a difference that would affect her future choice of stimuli for that client. Such experimental manipulations are easy to make during the course of treatment and allow the clinician to avoid making arbitrary assumptions without knowing their actual validity. This, of course, could not be accomplished adequately without accompanying objective information in the form of data obtained on line during treatment.

SUMMARIZING

Although the treatment described herein may sound very much like most clinicians' treatment, I have found that there are several critical differences between this version of operant conditioning and how clinicians typically design and execute treatment. One obvious difference is taking data during treatment. Further, although most clinicians have a natural sense of programming in terms of beginning with simple behaviors and gradually building upon them, this is usually not done with the precision suggested by programmed instruction, thus sometimes leaving some rather large or illogical gaps in the sequence of behaviors required of the client.

The major difference between typical clinical treatment and operant conditioning therapy, however, turns out to be what should be the simplest and most obvious principle of learning: the use of consequences. Although most clinicians appreciate that it is important to give clients feedback about the quality of their responses, most do this only very sloppily and much too infrequently. Further, they often make assumptions about the power of the stimuli they select as reinforcers and punishers that are not borne out by the data. Not only do clinicians pay too little attention to the selection of functional positive reinforcers and punishers, but they also fail to provide them regularly enough, immediately enough, or accurately enough. Learning is controlled primarily by events that *follow* responses. If a functional positive reinforcer is not provided often enough to establish a new behavior, the response will be extinguished. If a correct response is followed by a stimulus that is not a powerful reinforcer for the subject, or if the reinforcer is too delayed in its presentation, the correct response will be extinguished. If, conversely, a functional positive reinforcer is presented, but for a response that is "not quite right," then that same response will continue to occur because it has been reinforced. Therefore, I concentrate on selecting functional reinforcers and punishers and on presenting them immediately following correct and incorrect responses, respectively.

One last thing that I concentrate on during therapy: treatment time is the *client's* learning time. An operant philosophy dictates that clients learn by doing. Therefore, if I am hoarding treatment time by filling it with my own talking, the client has less opportunity to learn. The object of treatment is to present relevant stimuli to evoke appropriate responses and to arrange for their consequation. Evoking and consequating stimuli speak clearly enough for themselves; the client does not require much explanation from me in order to figure out what is desired of him. Within limits, the more time the client spends responding, the more learning is likely to occur.

SELECTED REFERENCES

Costello, J. Programmed instruction. *Journal of Speech and Hearing Disorders,* 1977, *42*:3-28.

Costello, J. Clinicians and researchers: A necessary dichotomy? *Journal of the National Student Speech and Hearing Association,* 1979, *7*:6-26.

Costello, J., and Ferrer, J. Punishment contingencies for the reduction of incorrect responses during articulation instruction. *Journal of Communication Disorders,* 1976, *9*:43-61.

Miller, K. *Principles of Everyday Behavior Analysis.* Monterey, CA: Brooks/Cole, 1980.

Stokes, T., and Baer, D. An implicit technology of generalization. *Journal of Applied Behavioral Analysis.* 1977, *10*:349-367.

CHAPTER TWO

TECHNIQUES OF THERAPY BASED ON MOTOR LEARNING THEORY

Method of Raymond D. Kent and John T. Lybolt

MOTOR SCHEMA AS A BASIS FOR MOTOR LEARNING

We take as a point of departure the premise that a motor skill is learned by establishing a *schema* which encodes movement targets and necessary feedback loops for coordination and error detection. A schema is a constructive and generalized relationship that is the foundation of all skilled motor behavior. It cannot be stressed too strongly that *a set of relationships* must be learned to acquire a motor skill. These relationships are summarized in Table 1 and include knowledge or perception of the goal, previous motor experience, ability to predict the sensory consequences of an action, and various decision mechanisms.

To understand what a schema is, it is important to recognize that a motor skill is not simply a motor action that is performed repeatedly with exactly the same set of movements in each performance. Rather, a motor skill is by its nature flexible and adaptive, so that each performance differs in some respect from every other performance. The movements in a particular instance of a motor skill are adjusted to the individual conditions that pertain to a given time. The notion of a schema is that motor performance is guided by the various factors listed in Table 1. Once the desired objective, or goal, is specified, the instantaneous conditions (current conditions and movements in progress) of the motor system are determined. In other words, the schema starts with information about (1) *what has to be done* and (2) *what the muscles are doing right now or have just completed doing*. Then the schema uses its storehouse of experience to determine *what it has done in the past when confronted with information (1) and (2) above*. From this previous motor experience, the schema generates the appropriate motor response, interpolating if necessary to generate a novel response to satisfy these special conditions.

The schema also generates the expected sensory consequences (feedback) for the motor act to be performed, that is, *what the*

TABLE 1 Fundamental Relationships Involved in Acquisition, Maintenance, and Performance of a Motor Skill

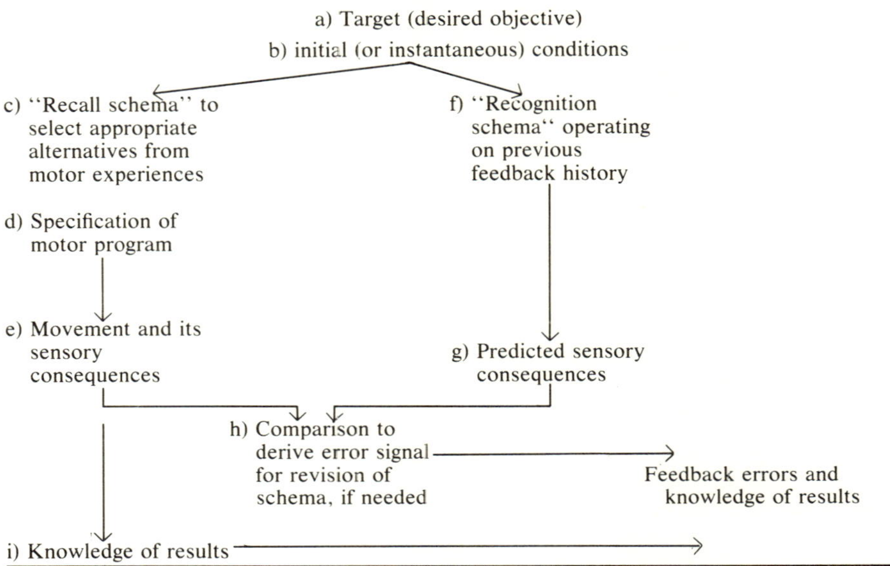

feedback should be. The *expected* sensory consequences are compared against the *actual* sensory consequences to derive an error signal. The error signal is used to adjust and refine the schema. In this way, the schema is gradually refined until it can cope with many variations in goals and instantaneous conditions.

One advantage of the schema theory of motor learning is that it can account for learning by trial-and-error and learning that is accomplished without knowledge of results. The schema also accounts for the so-called "novelty" problem—the fact that when we closely examine the movements associated with repeated performances of the same motor skill, the movements are not identical. Finally, schema theory helps to explain how neuromotor information necessary for speech can be stored and executed efficiently.

For any motor skill, including the motor skill component of speech, certain critical relationships must be developed and refined so that the motor behavior can be fluently adapted to differing conditions of performance. To take an example from the learning of speech sounds, an individual sound must be learned so that it can be produced easily and quickly in a variety of phonetic contexts. What we perceive as a given phoneme, like /k/ or /t/, is in fact a family of articulations. Because speech sounds are adapted to the phonetic context in which they occur, speech is not learned simply by acquiring knowledge of one articulatory position or one set of movement patterns for each phoneme in the language. Although each sound can be associated with a rather abstract description of its articulatory goal or target, the actual motor performance of speech is based on a complex and variable relationship between the abstract goal and the observable articulation. The abstract goal and the set of relationships linking it to the observable articulation schema gives us a motor learning perspective on the acquisition of speech sounds and on the management of "functional" misarticulations.

We can similarly conceptualize the situation faced by clients with dysarthria, dyspraxia, or fluency disorders. For an adult dysarthric speaker, the abstract goal has been established, but the client's access to sensory information about the current status of the articulators, or the results of a movement, may be limited. Furthermore, the adult dysarthric usually has lost the full capability of executing a motor program prepared by the schema. Dysarthric children often experience serious difficulties even in establishing the basic schema for speech. Because of impairments in motor performance and deficits in the monitoring and integration of sensory feedback, these clients may have poorly established schemata. Schema theory, with its emphasis on the integrated nature of the abstract goal of movement and the feedback loops involved in initiation, production, and error detection, helps us to conceptualize the difficulty faced by the dysarthric client. It also helps us to understand the reasons behind successful therapeutic techniques such as slowed rate, overarticulation, biofeedback training, syllable-by-syllable production, and efficient breath support for speech.

In the dyspraxic client, the fault may lie with the schema itself or with the mechanisms that support and execute the motor program. We believe that there are at least two or three types of dyspraxic disturbances, each affecting primarily a different aspect of the motor control process. Therapeutic techniques such as prosodic variation, feedback alteration or supplementation, and pacing are describable and understandable by the principles of motor schema theory.

Current research points to difficulty in moment-to-moment adjustments of the speech mechanisms as a fundamental disorder in stuttering. During fluent speech, stutterers display differences from normal kinematic parameters as well as differences in the synchrony of these parameters. Likewise, alterations of respiratory-laryngeal timing have been recorded. A variety of conditions induce fluency, and many of these directly alter the movements in stutterers' fluent speech. If stutterers' motor patterns are more variable than those of normal speakers, stutterers may encounter difficulties in sensing instantaneous conditions, deriving feedback for evolving movements, and computing error signals based on expected sensory consequences. Thus, procedures that lengthen the sampling time for movement control will promote speech fluency and are interpretable by the principles of schema theory.

SPECIAL TRAINING CONDITIONS

We often find it useful to apply special conditions to various phases of motor learning. Because these conditions are used at various times, from early training to final steps in transfer and generalization, it is most convenient to describe them now and refer to them as needed in the remainder of the chapter. Although we emphasize here the applications to management, these conditions also have value in diagnosis and assessment.

Bite block. A bite block is any object that can be inserted between the molars on either side of the jaw without risk of accidental swallowing. It is possible to fix the client's jaw opening at different distances by using bite blocks of different sizes. Because the jaw is the primary skeletal support for the tongue and lower lip, both lingual and labial articulations have to be adjusted as jaw position is varied. Thus, a bite block can be used to introduce articulatory modifications in the production of these sounds. We also use the bite block to evaluate and train articulatory function in subjects who seem to rely excessively on jaw movement to assist lingual and labial articulations. The bite block can be helpful when jaw stabilization is required to facilitate lingual or labial articulations.

Masking and Delayed Auditory Feedback Both of these feedback-altering conditions are useful in managing articulation disorders. Masking eliminates or reduces the auditory feedback available to the client and forces him or her to rely on other sources of feedback, such as taction and movement. If the masking noise is delivered to the client by headphones, with a good fit around the ears, the client's acoustic signal is still available to the clinician when it is masked to the client. Delayed auditory feedback (DAF) can be used similarly to alter a client's reliance on auditory feedback in the regulation of speech. By producing a slowed rate and at the same time increasing phonation time, DAF gives the client a greater opportunity to sample and interpret instantaneous feedback.

Rate, Stress, or other Prosodic Variations. We often rely on variation of prosodic aspects (speaking rate, stress, juncture, and intonation) to introduce and stabilize motor patterns. Whereas a slow-rate and heavy-stress condition is best suited to the early stages of learning, faster pace and reduced stress are aids to generalization and transfer. A primary effect of rate and stress is on the duration of a sound. When we want to maximize the feedback for a sound, we work with the sound in a slow-rate, heavy-stress condition to ensure an extensive articulatory movement for the sound and a long duration of articulatory positioning (and auditory feedback) for the sound. When we want to alter the feedback associated with a sound, we work with a faster speaking rate and varying degrees of stress. Other prosodic changes can be used in similar fashion. If we want to minimize a client's attention to auditory feedback for a given sound, we ask him or her to imitate very carefully our productions of prosodically varied passages, each of which contains one or more tokens of the sounds to be trained. This method diverts the client's attention from the individual sound to prosodic variation of a larger sequence. Pacing, or timekeeping imposed by an external device or nonspeech motor system, is another variant of a rate-modifying procedure. Particularly for clients with dyspraxia or fluency disorders, it can be helpful to assist the flow of speech with some rhythmic standard such as hand tapping.

Phonetic Context. There are indications from both clinical experience and formal research that production of a given sound can be influenced by its phonetic context, especially by the immediately preceding and following segments. Word and syllable position also appears to be a significant factor in selection of facilitating contexts for sound production. The principles to be used in selecting facilitating contexts are too involved to be summarized here, and so we refer the reader to a summary paper by R. Kent (Contextual Facilitation of Correct Sound Production) in *Language, Speech and Hearing Services in Schools*. Manipulation of phonetic context is useful not only to promote correct production of an error sound in early training, but also to ensure that practice items provide a wide range of articulatory-phonetic environments in which motor planning and feedback are sufficiently diverse. Thus, we consider phonetic context not only because we wish to discover contexts that facilitate correct production in an individual client, but also because phonetic context can be varied systematically to help establish the motor skills of interest.

SPECIFYING THE GOAL OR TARGET: DISCRIMINATION AND IMITATION TRAINING

The first requirement is adequate specification of the desired outcome—the *goal* or *target*. The basic objective is to specify the stimulus adequately so that the client is not hindered by uncertainties about the intended acoustic quality, articulatory position, range of movement, and so on. Of course, not all information about the goal or target will be immediately accessible to the client, as some information about the movement and its goal can be learned only through appropriate motor responses by the client. Studies of motor skill learning have shown that passive positioning of limbs, as through manipulation by a therapist, is not as successful in teaching a motor behavior as the client's own active participation in seeking proper positions and movements. To be certain that the goal or target is adequately understood by the client, we rely on auditory discrimination training, non-speech movements similar to the desired speech movement, visual information about the intended position or movement, and speech movements within the client's repertoire that are similar to the task or goal to be learned.

In *auditory discrimination training,* we follow the common procedure of asking the client to identify the sound to be trained in different contexts, proceeding from isolated production to production in a nonce monosyllable to production in phrases or sentences. Several commercially available auditory discrimination training programs can be used if a need for training is indicated. One of these, the Auditory Discrimination in Depth approach, focuses a client's attention on the motor precursors of the acoustically correct production. We have used this method successfully when children with serious articulation deficits have difficulty in transferring from single-word productions to more spontaneous productions. But the most important aspect of auditory discrimination is whether the client can use it to evaluate and modify his/her own articulatory responses. For this reason, we move quickly from discrimination tasks to imitation tasks, in which the client imitates a variety of sound patterns, including some that are not part of the English phonetic system.

Instructions given to modify motor behavior should relate as directly as possible to their performance by the client. This means that when we try to modify articulation, we use words that implement articulatory action, such as the following:

1. Your tongue is too low. Raise it up, like this (demonstrate, using, if appropriate, a related sound that the client produces correctly).
2. Your lips are too rounded. Hold them like this (demonstrate).
3. Close your jaw more when you say the sound.

We use such articulatory-based instructions in preference to comments like, "No, that doesn't sound right," or "It sounds too flat," or "That sounds more like a *w* than an *r*." Describing articulation in purely acoustic or auditory terms can be too abstract for the client's interpretation.

The schema theory has several implications for learning a new sound or other speech behavior. Our schema-based view of motor learning assumes that the motor commands (movement specifications generated by the brain) are selected in accord with both the goal and the instantaneous conditions of the articulators. From these two sources of information, a motor program is formulated by appropriate selection of previously learned motor commands. But what if no previously learned motor commands are fitted to the goal and the current conditions? It is in meeting exactly this need that schema theory has an advantage over other conceptions of motor learning. *We suppose that the schema, once it is sufficiently developed, can interpolate from its store of experience-based motor commands to derive commands that are tailored to the special, even unique, demands of a given situation.* Thus, previous motor experience will always influence the learning of a new skill or target. A motor behavior is not learned outside a person's perceptual-motor experience. A new speech sound is not learned without drawing on the client's previous motor patterns of sound production—whether intentionally or unintentionally. The influence of previous motor behavior at times is apparently negative, as when a client persistently draws on an older motor pattern that is unsuited to the behavior that is to be learned.

Imitation draws on the client's ability to formulate motor responses that are not necessarily in his practiced repertoire. A successful imitation requires that the client identify the relevant acoustic properties of the stimulus, select or formulate motor responses appropriate to reproduce the stimulus, and, finally, execute the motor plan. Imitative exercises with non-English sounds help to evaluate and train a client's imitative ability. Imitation draws on several abilities and is therefore useful in evaluating a client's ability to integrate auditory discrimination, response selection (or formulation), motor execution, and feedback appraisal.

All motor behavior produces *feedback,* or information about the motor act. In the case of speech, the client receives feedback from taction, position, movement, and audition. We believe that a major component of learning a motor skill is being able to predict the sensory consequences, or feedback, associated with it. For it is through the comparison of predicted and actual sensory consequences that a person can derive error information by which the schema can be revised and strengthened.

In the case of articulation training, we introduce the target or goal either in isolation or in small units such as monosyllable words or nonce syllables. For example, /s/ is attempted in isolation or in simple contexts (like a monosyllable) before it is worked into polysyllabic words or sentences. An overly complex context can interfere not only with response selection but also with effective focus on feedback. A complex context of movements can contaminate and confound the client's feedback for the behavior to be introduced or corrected. However, we believe that it is a mistake to linger too long on repetitive drills in which the same basic behavior is tediously practiced, to be followed by more tedious practice on another behavior. Not only is rote practice uninspiring to client and therapist, but research on motor skill learning shows that rote repetitive drill is much less successful than practice that constantly challenges by changing conditions. By analogy, one does not become an expert tennis player by attempting to use exactly the same stroke day after day. *Proficiency results from motoric adaptations to changing conditions.*

Among the reasons why we believe that repetitive production of isolated sounds is not an efficient approach to motor learning is that such practice does not yield the numerous and varied internal error signals that contribute to skill acquisition. Furthermore, isolated production does not give enough information on how a target can be reached from *different* starting positions and how a given target can be embedded in *different sequences* of motor responses.

Therefore, we emphasize *variability of practice,* not rote practice. Some authors distinguish acquisition and automatization by noting that acquisition involves perceptual elements and deliberate practice, whereas automatization involves extended practice under varying conditions. However, we believe that a skill is not acquired in a real sense without practice under varying conditions. To take acquisition of a speech sound as an example, we believe that the acquisition phase is accomplished by production of the sound in phonetically diverse contexts of short size, such as syllables, words, and brief phrases. Automatization is a phase in which the sound is produced in long and complex contexts. The objective of the acquisition phase is to establish the basic nature of the skill, or to establish the schema. The objective of the automatization phase is to produce the desired response under conditions of reduced attention and reduced or varied feedback.

Because of coarticulation, or the mutual influence that neighboring sounds exert on one another, and because normal speech production seems to be regulated in many ways by syllable-sized units, we prefer the syllable as a basic form for the manipulation of context. Many allophonic variations can be described with respect to position in a syllable (or alternatively as prevocalic or postvocalic forms). Although many sounds appear first in the normal developmental sequence as syllable-initial sounds, this result does not mean that the clinician should attempt to work with all misarticulated sounds in this position. Developmental evidence shows that the syllable-final position may be of advantage to certain sound classes such as fricatives. In addition, the final position is helpful in giving the client a lingering auditory, tactile, and kinesthetic feedback for the sound in training. Sounds in initial position often seem to have the relevant feedback "erased" by the influence of following sounds.

In addition, auditory feedback may be too slow for rapid error correction. More immediate feedback can be derived from tactile, positional, and movement cues. Even the ongoing movement generates some kinesthetic feedback, whereas auditory feedback sometimes is not available until after a position or movement has been achieved.

Whenever possible, we try to establish new or target behaviors in both syllable-initial and syllable-final positions, not only because this manipulation strengthens the schema, but also because it increases the number of linguistic forms to which generalization can occur. We also introduce rate and articulatory modifications to strengthen the schema and to vary the combination of relevant feedback signals. For example, once a sound is correctly articulated in a simple word such as *see* or *house,* we train for correct production in a task of maximum repetition rate for that syllable. If a client can articulate the sound correctly only under conditions of extreme prolongation, then he or she may be relying on slow-loop feedback (like audition) to regulate the articulation. Manipulation of rate of production can help to reduce the client's emphasis on slow-loop feedback channels. Another technique that may prove useful in establishing a motor pattern or feedback channel is to alter the conditions of articulation, as by asking the client to produce the sound as a bite block is used to control the amount of jaw lowering. Thus, the client is asked to produce the trained sound when the jaw is elevated (nearly closed), in mid-position, or extremely lowered (wide open).

One reason for the bite-block procedure is to force the client to produce the trained sound under greatly different articulatory conditions. The result is that the sound must be produced by positions and movements different from those by which it was originally elicited. The client thus experiences a different quality of feedback (at least at the tactile and kinesthetic levels), and has to produce the desired position or movement with a different combination of muscle activation.

Phonetic context can be used to meet essentially the same purposes, particularly if the therapist can identify contexts that are nonfacilitatory to production of the trained sound. Although the published reports on so-called facilitating phonetic contexts do not give us a complete picture about the basis for facilitation and the criteria by which facilitating or nonfacilitating contexts can be identified, we believe that phonetic contexts are not equal in eliciting correct production of an inconsistently articulated sound. Certain contexts seem to be preferable to others in obtaining a correct production. As noted by Kent (Contextual Facilitation of Correct Sound Production), both productive and perceptual factors can contribute to the judged facilitation provided by contextual manipulation, but the perceptual factors seldom have been studied. A review of the published studies on facilitation indicates that factors to be considered in the selection of initial contexts for sound training include syllable stress, word or syllable position, expected or permissible allophonic variation, frequency of occurrence, and the phonetic properties of surrounding sounds. (See the cited article for an analysis of these factors and for particular suggestions regarding the selection of facilitating contexts for /s/ and /r/.)

TRANSFER AND GENERALIZATION

Although acquisition, automatization, transfer, and generalization are often discussed as though they were independent phases of speech motor training, we think that it is important to emphasize that they are not independent. Motor schema theory implies that in motor speech training, rules or principles are stored, and these principles govern relationships among a person's knowledge or perception of the motor goal, previous motor experience, predictions of the sensory consequences of an action, and decision or control loops for carrying out the action and for error detection. If suggestions in the previous pages for the *acquisition phase* were followed, a rich foundation has already been laid for automatization, transfer, and generalization of the motor schema.

We actively assist clients in achieving transfer or an awareness of the motor schema for speech sound production in different contexts. This is done by providing an environment in which multiple correct responses can occur. Modeling and imitation trials across graded production levels, use of facilitating phonetic contexts, verbal instruction and feedback, and special training conditions, as discussed earlier, are used to give the child opportunities for productions in systematically varied contexts. Auditory discrimination training to help a child discern differences in his or her own acceptable and unacceptable productions is used when appropriate. Thus, attention is focused on perception of the motor goal, on the sensory consequences of the acceptable and unacceptable productions, and on pertinent aspects of the production for the development of motor control and feedback loops. Descriptions of successful transfer programs for stuttering emphasize the importance of providing more than "practice of oral motor behavior" that is free of stuttering. We agree with this concept, and by carefully controlling the duration, topic, and listener in a transfer trial, we try to provide the most facilitating conditions for a successful motor response. It is important that both the client's and clinician's estimate of potentially facilitating conditions be included in the transfer procedures.

Varying the incentive for motor speech changes is also important in achieving transfer of the desired motor response. Motor schema theory emphasizes that movement outcome is important in establishing and maintaining motor schemata. In treatment, we establish situations in which information is ineffectively transmitted unless the appropriate motor target is produced. Traditionally, minimal pairs have been used at this stage of acquisition training, and we have found this approach to be helpful. Motor schema theory would imply that alerting the child to important and salient aspects of the motor act is helpful. With younger children this is done using tactile or visual signaling, whereas older children may benefit from verbal cues as well ("Move your lips slowly"). A pause before the production for rehearsal, using cues given by the clinician, can be useful when transferring a motor speech act to a new context. "Blind communication tasks" in which the child's or the clinician's behavior is directly affected by the speech production are useful (For example, CHILD: "You get /θæm/." CLINICIAN: "What? I don't see /θæm/." CHILD: "You get /sæm/.") We also use a core vocabulary of words that are used frequently by the child and conform to the requirements of the transferred contexts. The clinician or parent "misunderstands" these vocabulary items if the child's productions are in error, and then models the correct and incorrect alternatives to help focus the child on the controlling properties of the appropriate motor target. Providing multiple opportunities for the child to convey pertinent, nonredundant, important information using the appropriate motor target is important in achieving transfer.

Generalization of highly practiced behavior to situations outside the therapy setting requires that the behavior not be a drain on cognitive or attention mechanisms. Motor behaviors established via the artificial communication typical of therapy sessions must be supplemented with a specific generalization program. Several factors that enhance generalization can be built into a program:

1. Follow-Through: Provide opportunities for the behavior to occur in appropriate contexts outside the establishment paradigm.
2. Self-Attribution: As appropriate for chronologic age, ensure that

the child is aware of the motor control that he exerts over his responding behavior (that his responses are not merely echoes of the clinician's model).

3. Self-Evaluation: Systematic self-evaluation of both perceptual motor and information transfer performance is taught; self-instruction/self-reinforcement assists with error detection.
4. Natural Environment: The treatment setting should not be so distinctively different from a normal communication setting that the motor speech behavior being taught is associated only with the former; begin to generalize transferred contexts as soon as possible.
5. Bridge with teachers and parents: Parents and teachers can provide a constant background of expectation for effective communication.

In our approach, as transfer to successive contexts through graded stimuli and production shifts occur, generalization of the originally transferred contexts can begin. Family members and teachers are alerted to expect certain productions, and to provide consistent situations for the speech behaviors to occur in relatively controlled manners. As new contexts are transferred, these are added to the generalization program, and the child is expected to monitor the appropriateness of those productions. In that portion of treatment not devoted to acquisition and automatization, previously transferred behaviors are elicited in natural communication settings. By limiting the number and the frequency of occurrence of speech acts in the generalization program, the clinician helps to ensure that cognitive and attentional demands are not such that the child is overwhelmed. In many communication disorders, speech motor performance can

TABLE 2 Suggested Factors for Consideration in Management of Individual Clients.

Phonetic context
Speaking rate
Prosodic content
Availability of feedback
Linguistic familiarity of stimuli
Restrictions on articulatory capability (e.g., bite block)
Emotional weight
Linguistic complexity
Familiarity of situation
Familiarity of topic
Listener's reaction
Informational impact
Client's concentration on selected aspects of communicative task

Generally, each of these factors can be varied or controlled to suit a management objective. For example, in making decisions about transfer and generalization, we consider how these factors might be used individually and in combination to achieve the desired result.

be influenced by the client's familiarity with a discussion topic, the syntactic complexity of modeled or required utterances, and the emotional weight of a situation or topic. All of these factors, then, are candidates for manipulation in a generalization program.

In making management decisions for any client, we consider several factors that might be used in the various phases of motor learning. A list of factors is present in Table 2. Not all of these factors are necessarily used for any given client, nor is this list exhaustive. The listed items simply represent some controllable aspects of the management setting, and they lend themselves to incorporation in a motor learning approach. To ensure that a client is capable of adaptive and flexible use of a learned motor response, we might begin the training or management process with manipulation of the first six variables in Table 2. That is, we would proceed with a program that is designed to train and evaluate production of the desired response across variations in phonetic context, rate, prosody, feedback availability, linguistic familiarity, and articulatory flexibility. These same factors are also applied in the transfer and generalization phases of training, but we add to them the other factors of emotional weight, linguistic complexity, familiarity of situation or topic, listener's reaction, informational impact, and directed concentration on the part of the client. In the earliest stages, it may be enough to introduce changes in only one factor, such as phonetic context. In the latest stages, we introduce concomitant changes in several variables, to increase the cognitive demands of the task and thus alter the client's feedback and attentional strategies.

SELECTED REFERENCES

Kent, R. Contextual facilitation of correct sound production. *Language, Speech and Hearing Services in Schools*, 1982, *13*:66-76.

Marteniuk, R. Cognitive information processes in motor short-term memory and movement production. In G. E. Stelmach (Ed.), *Motor Control: Issues and Trends*. New York: Academic Press, 1976, pp. 175-186.

Schmidt, R. The schema as a solution to some persistent problems in motor learning theory. In G. Stelmach (Ed.), *Motor Control: Issues and Trends*. New York: Academic Press, 1976, pp. 41-65.

Semjen, A. From motor learning to sensorimotor skill acquisition. *Journal of Human Movement Studies*, 1977, *3*:182-191.

Shelton, R., and McReynolds, L. Functional articulation disorders: Preliminaries to treatment. In N. Lass (Ed.), *Speech and Language: Advances in Basic Research and Practice, Vol. 2*. New York: Academic Press, 1979.

CHAPTER THREE

TECHNIQUES OF THERAPY BASED ON CLASSICAL CONDITIONING

Method of C. Woodruff Starkweather

The basic paradigm for classical conditioning is

$$S_1 \longrightarrow S_2$$

in which S_1 = a conditioned stimulus, or CS, and S_2 = an unconditioned stimulus, or UcS. The arrow means that S_2 will occur only if S_1 occurs; S_2 is contingent on S_1.

An unconditioned stimulus (S_2) is defined as any stimulus with a valence that is not neutral. The valence of a stimulus refers to the attitude a person has toward it. Valence may be identified by observing the person's reaction to the stimulus. Stimuli with negative valence (S^-) are aversive; they provoke pain, discomfort, fear, or any unpleasant reaction, mild or severe. People avoid them. Stimuli with positive valence (S^+) are pleasant or enjoyable, and people approach them, stay near them, or interact with them. Whether positive or negative, the reaction to an unconditioned stimulus is reliable. That reaction is called the unconditioned response, or UcR.

A conditioned stimulus (S_1) is defined as a stimulus with a neutral valence (S^0). The conditioned stimulus provokes no particular attitude or reaction. It is neither positive nor negative.

When S_2 is contingent on S_1, and when a person repeatedly experiences this pairing of the two stimuli, classical conditioning occurs. The effect of classical conditioning is to create an attitude toward or reaction to S_1 that is similar to the reaction that previously occurred to S_2. In other words, a conditioned response to the S_1 develops, which is similar to the unconditioned response to the S_2.

For example, a client who continually fails (S_2^-) in school may learn to fear certain teachers, classes, subjects, or the physical settings (S_1's) that have been systematically associated ($S_1 \longrightarrow S_2^-$) with the experience of failure. If the emotional reaction happens also to produce a speech disorder, such as dysphonia, the client will become dysphonic when he is talking to those teachers, in those classes, or about those subjects in which failures occurred. Therapy will be constructed so as to decondition, countercondition, or desensitize the client to these specific stimuli. On the positive side, a clinician who constructs therapy plans carefully so that each step in therapy challenges the client at a level where he can succeed will find that the therapy setting, the clinician, and the process of working on speech or language are all S_1's that have acquired a positive valence because they were systematically associated ($S_1 \longrightarrow S_2^+$) with the positive experience of achievement (S_2^+). Clients who have been conditioned in this way will work because they enjoy it.

It is through classical conditioning that we acquire attitudes and learn to like or dislike things. Because of this, classical conditioning often determines what stimuli can be used as reinforcers or punishers in instrumental conditioning. Although some stimuli are inherently pleasant (food, sex) or aversive (pain), most ordinary stimuli such as activities, settings, or people have an acquired valence. We like or dislike them because of the experiences we have had with them. It is these stimuli that are the reinforcers or punishers of everyday behavior. And since our experience is continuously accumulating, what is reinforcing one day may not be reinforcing the next. It is often overlooked that instrumental behavior is determined primarily by the current conditions of reinforcement and nonreinforcement and only weakly by the influence of past conditions. Changing the valence of a reinforcer for some instrumentally conditioned behavior is as effective an extinction procedure as withdrawing the stimulus. Classical conditioning thus plays an important part in maintaining instrumentally conditioned behavior.

Suppose that a child with several phonologic substitutions has learned in therapy enough correct phonologic behavior so that he is able to speak intelligibly. The new behaviors are now being transferred to outside situations. One of the reinforcers might be the additional scholastic success his new way of talking brings him. But the positive feeling these successful experiences give him depends on an association between scholastic achievement and other positive feelings, such as admiration from peers or parents. If the child starts to be influenced by some new friends who scoff at schoolwork, the positive valence of achievement will diminish, and its reinforcement value will decline.

Before attempting to transfer a newly acquired behavior into a client's everyday life, I try to find out what his likes and dislikes are. I construct practice assignments so that the new behavior will be instrumental in helping him achieve desirable things and avoid undesirable ones. If there is little opportunity for his improved speech to help him achieve reinforcement, which is often the case, I try to arrange for the child to develop an interest in some activity where his better speech will bring him admiration from peers or parents. Development of a new interest is a job for classical conditioning. Clinicians arrange the situation so that the things they want the client to like (S_1) are frequently associated with the things he already likes (S_2^+).

Self-reinforcement—the feeling of pride in any successful achievement— is probably also first learned by classical conditioning as parents react with delight, amusement, affection, and attention to a child's first accomplishments. But self-reinforcement needs an occasional booster shot in the form of attention from parents or significant other people. The classical conditioning needs to be kept current. I try to involve parents and teachers, and, whenever feasible, siblings and friends, in a client's therapy. However, it is usually a mistake to tell other people, even parents, to give the child a pat on the head when they hear him use the correct speech behavior. If the parents, teachers, and friends are aware that the client is working on a particular behavior, they will react to his correct productions with a show of approval that is natural for that client. This one demonstration will boost the client's own feelings of accomplishment, which will help to self-reinforce the next few behaviors.

Classical conditioning may also be directly involved in the acquisition or maintenance of fluency and vocal behavior. These two aspects of communicative behavior seem more susceptible to emotion than others. Under stress, prosody often changes. And emotion, most particularly stress, is often said to disrupt fluency and clear vocal tone. Consequently, therapies for stuttering and voice disorders make use of three techniques derived from classical conditioning: deconditioning, counterconditioning, and desensitization.

Deconditioning is the extinction process for classically conditioned behavior. Extinction occurs when the CS (S_1) is experienced, but the UcS (S_2) is not, so that the two stimuli are disassociated:

$$S_1 \longrightarrow \emptyset.$$

As a result, the previously acquired attitude toward the S_1 diminishes; its valence is neutralized. With repeated $S_1 \longrightarrow \emptyset$ experiences, S_1 will regain the neutral valence it had before conditioning took place. For example, during times of family crisis, such as a serious illness, a large proportion of telephone calls may be anxiety provoking. After a few such calls, we can be classically conditioned so that the ringing of the telephone makes our hearts beat faster and our hands get sweaty. We have learned to react to the ring of the phone (S_1) with behavior similar to that previously reserved for the bad news itself (S_2^-). After the crisis has passed, however, telephone calls become more balanced. Some are still unpleasant (S_2^-), but just as many are pleasant (S_2^+), and most are neutral (S_2^0). As a result, the ringing of the phone becomes disassociated from unpleasant news, and the fear reaction to it gradually subsides.

In counterconditioning, the neutralization of S_1 is helped along by the contingent presentation of stimuli having the opposite valence. Suppose that a series of $S_1 \longrightarrow S^-$ experiences have caused S_1 to have a negative valence. The effect can be countered by a series of $S_1 \longrightarrow S^+$ experiences. Consequently, a negative attitude or emotion toward a particular stimulus, such as a speech situation, word, or listener, can be neutralized by arranging for the stimulus to be associated with happy events.

To use deconditioning and counterconditioning in therapy, clinicians have to be able to rearrange the client's life a little, so that speech situations are associated less with negative and more often with positive stimuli. With children, the family's style of communication can often be changed, so that more $S_1 \longrightarrow S_2^+$ and $S_1 \longrightarrow S_2^0$ and fewer $S_1 \longrightarrow S_2^-$ events occur. I try to make sure that verbal competition, ridicule, and "demand speech" ("Tell your Aunt Corinne about the play") are eliminated. These situations make children afraid to talk. Fear can aggravate dysphonia and disfluency; it can slow word-retrieval time, and it can reduce syntactic complexity and utterance length. I tell the parents to make sure the child gets natural opportunities to talk without having to interrupt or shout other people down and that his contributions are accepted (not applauded) for whatever value they have according to the child's own level of performance. With adults, it's harder to rearrange speech situations so that they are less aversive. Instead, desensitization is used.

The term "desensitization" is commonly applied to procedures aimed at dealing with fear or anxiety. Two such procedures, quite different from each other, can be identified. In the first type, the client is encouraged, by persuasion or tangible incentives, to approach the feared stimulus, to confront it, or to become more familiar with it. The object is to toughen the client, to reduce his sensitivity to stimuli that are aversive to him. This is the type of desensitization used in nonavoidance therapies for stuttering. It is assumed that stutterers learn to fear certain words, listeners, and speech situations because they have often stuttered under these circumstances. Stuttering is presumed to be aversive. Confronting and becoming more familiar with stuttering reduces the client's sensitivity to it. Although it has been empirically demonstrated that increased familiarity with genuinely aversive stimuli weakens their aversiveness, this form of desensitization is widely used only in nonavoidance therapies for stuttering. The desensitization used in the treatment of functional dysphonia is typical of the other type.

I begin the first type of desensitization by demonstrating my own willingness to talk about stuttering, then to stutter myself, first in the clinic, then in outside situations. As the client becomes involved, he begins to contribute his own thoughts about *his* stuttering and his own demonstrations of behavior. The focus of discussion shifts from stuttering in general to *his* stuttering. Clinicians who find it uncomfortable to model stuttering may want to rely on a videotape library of other stutterers as a way of beginning this type of desensitization. Gradually, the client becomes more and more involved in learning about his stuttering and in teaching me about it. Forays into the real world to test ideas and gather information increase in frequency and difficulty. Usually, by this time real stuttering has greatly diminished and faked stuttering is used. When the client's fears of stuttering have been largely desensitized, according to his own report, I begin direct modification of stuttering behavior.

The initial desensitization phase of therapy is completed when the client reports feeling much less afraid in most of his difficult situations. However, as we begin the next phase, in which the stuttering behaviors themselves are removed, fears typically return or increase in severity, and a second phase of desensitization begins. This second phase of desensitization runs concurrently with direct modification of stuttering, and its goal is not the reduction of emotion but learning how to handle the emotions that occur during stuttering so that they do not disrupt speech behavior. As stutter-free speech via slow-motion transitions (both the pull-out and the preparatory set type) are practiced, the effects of rising emotion are examined and dealt with. By learning to pay attention to his speech behavior and the emotions that accompany it, as they are happening, the stutterer can learn to deal with both.

The second type of desensitization is most commonly associated with Wolpe's systematic desensitization. In this type, stimuli such as speech situations or difficult listeners provocative of disfluency or dysphonia are imagined in order from the least to the most feared. These scenes are typically imagined under induced relaxation in a protected environment where no aversive stimulation can occur. Consequently, the feared scene (S_1) is presented without its aversive consequences ($S_1 \longrightarrow \emptyset$) and is consequently deconditioned. It is also often said that the fear response is inhibited by the relaxation process since it is impossible to be relaxed and anxious at the same time. However, hierarchical presentation of feared stimuli, without relaxation, is an equally effective desensitization procedure, so probably the process involved is simple deconditioning.

Here's how it works. First, a hierarchy of the feared stimuli is constructed. This is simply a list of stimuli ranked according to how much fear they cause. Second, the client is trained in relaxation by progressive muscle relaxation, or by hypnotic suggestion, or by both. Once he can achieve a deep state of relaxation, he is asked to imagine the feared stimuli, beginning with those that are least disturbing and proceeding up the hierarchy. As the client imagines a scene, he signals (by raising a finger usually) if he feels any fear. When this happens, the scene is terminated by the clinician, the client is re-relaxed, and the scene re-presented. If, after several tries, the client still signals that the scene is disturbing, it can be re-presented in a weakened form. Once he is desensitized to the weaker form, the full-strength version is imagined again. The goal is three or four presentations of a stimulus without reaction. Then, it is time to move on up the hierarchy to the next stimulus situation. This continues until reactions to all stimuli have been desensitized. Systematic desensitization can be, and should be, combined with real-life experiences to validate the extent to which desensitization has actually occurred. Subjective client reports can be "quantified" using a Subjective Units of Disturbance (SUDS) scale, which varies from 0 (complete calm) to 100 (outright panic).

The success of systematic desensitization depends on a number of conditions, which particular clients may or may not meet. First, the fear reaction to the S_1 must be unrealistic, that is, the S_2 cannot be genuinely aversive. If it is, and if the $S_1 \longrightarrow S_2^-$ contingency persists in the client's every-day life, it will undo any deconditioning that takes place in the clinic. There are, however, ways of getting around this problem, such as in vivo desensitization and/or counterconditioning. Second, the client must be able to imagine the scenes vividly enough so that the imaginary scene approximates the real one, for the success of the procedure depends on generalization from imaginary to real events. Third, the client must cooperate by actually imagining what the clinician tells him to. He cannot get too creative or he may begin to imagine aversive events. Thus, clients must be imaginative enough, but not too imaginative.

Occasionally in systematic desensitization, positively valenced stimuli are imagined immediately after a feared scene is imagined ($S_1 \longrightarrow S_2^+$) to speed up or strengthen the neutralization process by counterconditioning. Systematic desensitization is used in the treatment of stuttering, functional dysphonia, and a variety of fear-related psychobehavioral disorders, including elective mutism, speech fear, and hysterical aphonia.

AVOIDANCE CONDITIONING

Although often called "instrumental avoidance conditioning," this process actually combines classical and instrumental conditioning in a special way. A signal (S_1) informs the client that if a certain behavior (R_1) is not performed, aversive events (S_2^-) will follow. Symbolically, it looks like this:

$$S_1 - R_1 \longrightarrow S_2^-$$

The minus sign means that given S_1, the absence of R_1 will result in S_2^-. Thus, R_1 is performed in order to avoid S_2^-. Avoidance conditioning is a common process in everyday life. We are often able to forestall aversive consequences; applying the brakes in a car as you approach a red light is an avoidance behavior. The combination of classical and instrumental processes is apparent from the fact that two events are required to result in S_2^-, the stimulus S_1 and the nonperformance of R_1. Elimination of either—i.e., the nonoccurrence of S_1 or the performance of R_1—means that S_2^- will not occur. Thus there is a double contingency: $S_1 \longrightarrow S_2$ and $(-R_1) \longrightarrow S_2^-$. The first is a classical (stimulus-contingent) and the second is an instrumental (response-contingent) type. As a result of avoidance conditioning, two things happen: (1) the valence of S_1 becomes more negative, which means that the client learns to react fearfully to it, and (2) the frequency of R_1 increases. However, as the client becomes more adept at performing the avoidance behavior (R_1), the negative emotional reaction to the stimulus (S_1) is likely to become subdued. The client becomes confident that the avoidance behavior is readily available as a way of forestalling the threatened aversive event, and so he has nothing to fear.

This process results in behavior with particular characteristics. First, the behavior may or may not appear to be fear-motivated, depending on how well-learned the avoidance response is. Second, any real threat may have disappeared, and yet the behavior persists. This is because during conditioning, when the threat was real, the response succeeded in averting it so that there were no aversive consequences. Later, even if the possibility of real aversive consequences no longer exists, extinction does not occur because when the client performs the avoidance behavior, nothing happens. Often, too, the original threat is imaginary, exaggerated, or modeled by others, but once the behavior has been acquired, such things do not matter. In a sense, the reality of the aversive consequences are confirmed for the client *because* they do not occur when the avoidance behavior is used. Typically, avoidance behavior occurs tenaciously, with or without any real threat, and a simple withdrawal of the contingency does little to extinguish it.

Extinction of avoidance behavior must deal with both the classical and the instrumental components. This is accomplished by a combination of (1) desensitizaion to S_2 by increased familiarity (type 1) or desensitization to S_1 through deconditioning (type 2) and (2) nonreinforcement of R_1 by response-prevention. Response-prevention consists of inducing the client not to perform the avoidance behavior, typically by reinforcing another behavior that is incompatible with it. The clearest example of this extinction process is in nonavoidance therapy for stutterers where desensitization to stuttering and feared speech situations is combined with the performance of controlled fluent speech gestures or voluntary stuttering, either of which prevent, by their incompatiblity with it, the habitual avoidance reaction.

I begin nonavoidance therapy with desensitization through familiarization. Then I introduce response-prevention techniques. As a result of the first desensitization phase, the client is familiar with his stuttering pattern, both the emotional and behavioral parts of it, and is accustomed to talking about it and demonstrating it. With the client's emotional reaction attenuated, stuttering behaviors are greatly reduced in frequency and severity. Those that remain are the targets of response-prevention. The client is asked to attend carefully to his stuttering while it is happening and to change the behavior so as to restore normally fluent, forward-moving speech. What kinds of changes he makes depend on the type and anatomical location of the stuttering. He might have to learn to loosen up laryngeal tension and begin voicing, or stop repeating a sound and say the rest of the word. In either of these two examples, the fluent behavior—voicing or saying the rest of the word—is incompatible with the stuttering behavior and prevents it from occurring. The difficulty is that the stuttering behaviors are well learned, and the presence of emotional reactions distracts the client from the task. For this reason, attending to emotions and keeping them from interfering is a secondary aspect of this modification phase. As the client begins to gain control over his feelings and speech, and can use fluent speech to prevent stuttering, situational practice, already begun in the earlier desensitization phase, continues for newly learned fluency behaviors. With continued practice in and out of the clinic, control over speech is regained. A maintenance phase then begins in which the frequency of therapy contacts is gradually reduced. If setbacks occur, the frequency of therapy is sometimes temporarily increased, then diminished again to maintenance level. Preparing the client in how to deal with temporary setbacks is an important part of the maintenance phase.

Other speech and language disorders may also be linked to avoidance conditioning. Certainly hysterical aphonia and elective mutism appear to be strategies adopted by clients to avoid penalties associated with talking. The case for conditioning is strengthened by the common clinical report that there is often in these clients a history of voicelessness or speechlessness which has previously been instrumental in avoiding some unpleasant experience. Another problem that may be attributed to avoidance conditioning is the language deficit often seen in stuttering children. These children may learn through avoidance-conditioning that using shorter sentences and fewer words, or even simpler syntactic structures, results in speech that is less disfluent. Advanced forms of hyperfunctional dysphonia may also be attributed to avoidance conditioning. Often, when the vocal mechanism is structurally inadequate because of injury, swollen through misuse, or burdened by the presence of a growth, clients find that the voice they can produce under these circumstances is unpleasant to them and to their listeners. Many of them begin to struggle with tension and force to produce a voice that they can live with. The struggling and tension is an avoidance behavior that is instrumental, or is thought to be instrumental, in producing a voice that is less aversive to the speaker. For any of these clients, techniques combining desensitization and response-prevention should be useful.

SELECTED REFERENCES

Bandura, A. *Principles of Behavior Modification*. New York: Holt, 1969.

Starkweather, C. A multiprocess behavioral approach to stuttering therapy. In W. Perkins, (Ed.), *Strategies in Stuttering Therapy*. A volume in the series Seminars in Speech, Language and Hearing. Edited by J. Northern. 1980, 1:327-338.

Starkweather, C. *Speech and Language: Principles and Process of Behavior Change*. Englewood Cliffs, N.J.: Prentice-Hall, 1982.

Wolpe, J. *The Practice of Behavior Therapy*. New York: Pergamon Press, 1969.

CHAPTER FOUR

TECHNIQUES OF THERAPY BASED ON COGNITIVE LEARNING THEORY

Method of C. Woodruff Starkweather

An important distinction in learning theory is between observable and unobservable behavior. Many behaviorists use "behavior" only in reference to observable activity, but this is too restrictive. No matter what it is called, unobservable behavior, especially cognitive behavior, is important in people's lives. A description of speech and language without reference to cognitive behavior would be empty. Indeed, it was the exclusion of cognitive events that made Skinner's descriptions of language behavior so paltry. Nevertheless, because cognitive behavior cannot be seen directly, care must be taken in making assumptions about the role these events play in speech and language.

A cognitive response is simply a thought or feeling, typically in reaction to some stimulus. But a thought or feeling may also serve as a stimulus for a subsequent response. So a cognitive event may act either as a stimulus or as a response, or as both, as these events often do.

Since both responses and stimuli may be covert, it is evident that the usual conditioning processes—instrumental (operant) conditioning, classical conditioning, avoidance conditioning—can take place with cognitive behavior or with combinations of cognitive and external behavior. Instrumentally conditioned cognitive behaviors are often called *coverants* to distinguish them from their observable cognates, operants. Specific conditioning and extinction procedures too—reinforcement, punishment, deconditioning, counterconditioning, desensitization, discrimination, and generalization—can take place with cognitive responses and stimuli. Another process—vicarious conditioning—has particular relevance to cognitive events, and will be discussed here.

CLASSICALLY CONDITIONED SEMANTIC BEHAVIOR

Although simple classical conditioning, described elsewhere in this volume, is most commonly thought of in connection with emotional or attitudinal learning, it also describes with great elegance and simplicity how a child can learn to understand the meanings of words. A person who knows the meaning of a word reacts cognitively in a certain way when he hears the word spoken. A child who has not yet learned the meaning of a word does not react this way. It is proposed that this change in cognitive reaction to the word is, or may be, classically conditioned. Suppose that a child does not yet know the meaning of the word *ball*. He still reacts with specific cognitive and perceptual behavior when he sees a ball. These behaviors occur reliably whenever the object is perceived. The object is thus a UcS (S_2) and the cognitive/perceptual events that occur in response to it constitute a UcR. The word, not yet learned, produces no such reaction and so qualifies as a CS (S_1). When the child hears the word used repeatedly at the same time he perceives the object or event it refers to, he begins to respond to the word with cognitive behavior that is similar (but not identical) to the behaviors previously caused by the perception of the object. The new cognitive response to the word corresponds roughly to the "idea" or "concept" of a category to which the object belongs. When first learned, of course, this "concept" is likely to be overspecified, possibly referring to only one object, and it is likely to be erroneous, too. In any event, the word is a CS, the object a UcS, and they are clearly in a contingent, or dependent, relationship. Thus, it is suggested that word comprehension may be learned by classical conditioning of the form

$$S_1 \longrightarrow S_2$$

where S_1 = a word, and S_2 = environmental events or objects representative of the word's meaning.

The kinds of errors a child makes when first using a word support this idea. These errors, which have been described in writings on semantic feature theory, suggest that what the word means to the child depends on what, in the child's experience, the word has been associated with. As the child's experience of these word-referent associations gradually approximates the experience of competent speakers, these errors drop out. The idea that word meanings may be learned by classical conditioning clarifies a number of other language-learning processes.

First, once the child has learned to comprehend some content words, these words reliably cause cognitive behavior themselves and can consequently serve as UcS's for the classical conditioning of additional word meanings. A meaningful word is as much a part of a person's experience as any other environmental event. As a result, the comprehension of relational terms, morphological markers, and other elements of language that depend for their meaning on other words can be acquired by the same classical conditioning process.

Second, phonologic rules may be learned along with word meanings. The complete proof for this assertion is too complex for inclusion here, but there is evidence that early phonologic rules are semantically related. As the child learns the meaning of a word, he of course learns what sounds it is composed of. With the learning of more words, certain phonemic features become distinctive because they contrast or differentiate words that have different meanings. The semantically contrastive system of phonemes is thus built up from a relatively small number of features. Phonologic rules prohibiting certain categories of sounds, certain combinations of sounds, and cerain distributions of sounds in a language are a result of the child's not having had any experiences in which he heard words containing these sounds and combinations being used meaningfully by competent speakers.

Third, the meanings of sentences, in which syntactic relations between words stand for environmental relations between events and objects, may also be acquired by classical conditioning. This is an idea that seems more acceptable when it is understood that both sentence structure and environmental relations have genuine stimulus value, that is, they are events to which discrete cognitive responses occur. Consequently, the meaning of a structural element can be acquired by classical conditioning in which the structural element is systematically associated with the relation it stands for. This is discussed later in this chapter.

Finally, each experience of a classical conditioning type, in which

$$S_1 \longrightarrow S_2$$

where S_1 = a language form, and S_2 = an aspect of experience the form represents (which may be responbsible for the acquisition of receptive language behavior) is at the same time an experience of vicarious conditioning (to be discussed) in which a competent speaker of the language models the expressive use of the same form. Consequently, the acquisition of language forms, in receptive and expressive modes, can be accounted for by the conditioning processes. Furthermore, by invoking the processes of generalization and discrimination, a more elaborate and refined theory of language behavior can be described with the well-known processes of learning. This has the distinct advantage of placing language acquisition within the same framework as language therapy.

The possibility that classical conditioning may be the process through which children learn the meanings of words and sentences has a number of therapeutic implications. First, and most clearly, clinicians interested in enriching the number of forms to which clients can respond appropriately will want to arrange therapeutic experiences of the form

$$S_1 \longrightarrow S_2$$

where S_1 = the form to be learned, and S_2 = an example of the referential category the form stands for.

The procedure is as follows:

1. Establish the forms that the child already knows. Two criteria should be met: consistency and generality. The consistency criterion is met if the child responds appropriately to the form when it is used to refer to exactly the same object/event on several different occasions. The generality criterion is met when the child responds appropriately to the form when it is used to refer to a reasonable variety of objects/events in the category the form represents. The word "reasonable" is used because some forms refer to a very large number of different objects/events, whereas others refer to much narrower categories. Also, the extent to which comprehension of a form is fully generalized within a category is an aspect of development.

2. From an understanding of the order in which forms are typically learned, establish a list of forms that should be targeted for therapy. Select among these the one that should be easiest to learn, considering ease of discrimination, salience of the referent, breadth of the category, and so on.

3. Present the form in a simple and natural but consistent sentence frame, such as "Look, a ______," for nouns referring to visible things. This should be done while the object/event to which the form refers is present physically or pictorially, *and the child is attending to it*. It takes clinical ingenuity to arrange activities and materials so that the child apprehends both the word and its referent in close association. Of course, it also presupposes a certain level of cognitive development in the child.

4. After several paired associations, test for comprehension of the form with the same object/event, but with a variation of the context. Often, the context needs to be altered gradually since children may erroneously associate elements of the context with the form, just as in natural language learning, particularly when the form is not particularly salient.

5. When the consistency criterion for one referent has been met, another example of the same referential category can be intro-

duced. Thus, each example reaches the consistency criterion before another one is introduced.

6. When a sufficient variety of examples seems to have been acquired, test for generality by seeing if the child responds to use of the form with a novel referent. When *several* novel referents result in appropriate responses to the form in a variety of contexts, the child can be said to understand its meaning.

7. Choose another form.

The process of classical conditioning may also be used to teach the meaningfulness of a syntactic structure by presenting the form in association with examples of environmental relations that the structure stands for. The procedural steps are the same as those given above for teaching word meanings, but the method for presenting a syntactic element in association with environmental relations will be different. Question forms, for example, can be modeled by the clinician, and the answer supplied by an aide. Although this is a vicarious conditioning process (to be discussed) for *expressive* use of the form, it is at the same time a classical conditioning technique for receptive use. The child watches a competent speaker using the question form (S_1). At the same time, the clinician/model provides nonverbal and situational cues that signal a search for information (S_2), thus associating the form with the event it stands for ($S_1 \longrightarrow S_2$). The answer supplied by the aide confirms the referent. As a general rule, the context, both the immediate environment and other accompanying language, can supply the stimulation (S_2) required to teach a new form. Again, criteria for consistency and generality should be met, but because the generality of a syntactic structure is broader than that of a word, a larger number of examples of the referent will need to be presented before the child will be able to abstract a rule and use it to understand new tokens of the same form.

COGNITIVE INSTRUMENTAL CONDITIONING

Consider a simple instrumental conditioning paradigm,

$$R_1 \longrightarrow S_1^+$$

in which a positively valenced stimulus is contingent on a response. Either or both of the elements in this contingency could be covert:

$$\bar{R}_1 \longrightarrow \bar{S}_1^+.$$

When a client discovers ($\bar{R}_1$), a principle the clinician is explaining or modeling, it gives a small feeling of accomplishment, satisfaction, or discovery ($\bar{S}_1^+$). In this case both the response and the reinforcer are covert. When, in addition to thinking about it, he actually uses the principle to generate a correct utterance (R_1), his feeling of accomplishment is enhanced ($\bar{S}_1^+$), and in this second case, the response is overt and the reinforcer covert. This is a common combination, but the opposite type—covert behavior with external reinforcement—cannot easily occur, since the covert behavior is not observable by others who would probably supply the reinforcement. Frequently, however, covert behavior ($\bar{R}_1$) results in an overt performance (R_2), which is externally reinforced, and the covert behavior participates in this reinforcement.

$$\bar{R}_1 + R_2 \longrightarrow S_1^+ .$$

Covert punishment ($\bar{R}_1 \longrightarrow \bar{S}_1^-$) and covert nonreinforcement ($\bar{R}_1 \longrightarrow \emptyset$)are two other types of cognitive instrumental conditioning processes.

When two people talk to each other, the intention of the speaker is a cognitive behavior ($\bar{R}_1$), which becomes public and overt (R_2) after it has been encoded. There is reinforcement value in communicating. This is evident from the fact that we communicate with great frequency and from experiments that demonstrate that we will perform other tasks in order to earn the opportunity to communicate. So, as a behavior, communication seems to be universally self-reinforcing, more like eating or sex than like learning to swing a golf club properly. Perhaps this self-reinforcement comes from the sharing of private experience. Certainly, those who cannot communicate suffer a terrible isolation.

Another aspect of talking is that it exerts powerful control over the cognitive behavior of listeners. Not that a speaker always achieves the control he desires, but speech creates an opportunity for control, which may be reinforcing itself or lead to subsequent reinforcement. Without speech and language this form of reinforcement is unavailable.

In short, language has many uses, and each use gains reinforcement for the language user. The broad usefulness of language is probably why people use it so much, which is simply another way of saying that the frequency of speech and language behavior is high because it is reinforced often.

Studies of language pragmatics specify the many uses of language. There are discriminative stimuli that signal when the use of a particular form is appropriate. When use is appropriate for the context, reinforcement is the successful communication of intention. When, given a certain context such as the relative status of speaker and listener, the appropriate form for the context is not used, the intention may not be correctly perceived, and a nonreinforcing failure of communication will result. Pragmatics is thus viewed as a form of instrumental behavior in which specific cues (S_1) signal that a specific form (R_1) will result in the successful communication of a speaker's intention (S_2^+):

$$S_1 + R_1 \longrightarrow S_2^+.$$

When the covert events are included.

$$S_1 + \bar{S}_2 + \bar{R}_1 + R_2 \longrightarrow S_3^+ \text{ (or } \bar{S}_3^+\text{)},$$

where S_1 = cue from context, $\bar{S}_2$ = cognitive events caused by the context, $\bar{R}_1$ = communicative intent, R_2 = overt communicative act, and S_3^+ (or $\bar{S}_3^+$) = overt (or covert) reinforcement from successful communication of intention.

Although the study of language pragmatics is relatively new, some suggestions have been made that certain clients may have both the intention to communicate and the language forms with which to express the intention, but still lack the pragmatic ability to use language properly.

Such clients may have adequate semantic and syntactic behavior, but have disordered pragmatic behavior. They would understand what forms mean and be able to construct and understand sentences, but choose forms that are inappropriate for the context, for example, on a formal occasion using informal language, or talking on the telephone without using the special forms that the nonvisual mode requires. Of course, children at certain stages of development do these things, and any conclusion about a disorder of pragmatics should be weighed against developmental norms, of which only some are known at present.

In any event, it is evident to me that discrimination training is the method by which pragmatic language behavior can be taught. The client is using a form that would be correct in other circumstances, but incorrect for the present context.

In discrimination training the clinician reinforces behavior that is contextually appropriate and, contrastively, does not reinforce the same behavior when performed in inappropriate contexts. Consequently the procedure is as follows:

1. Make a list of the contexts (S_1) in which forms are inappropriately used.

2. For each S_1, identify alternative contexts (S_2) in which the same forms would be appropriate.

3. Present each pair of S_1's and matching S_2's in a sequence designed to heighten the contrast between them, reinforcing the client for appropriate behavior only. There are four possible combinations of context and behavior, two of which generate reinforcement and two of which do not:

$$S_1 + R_1 \longrightarrow S^+$$
$$S_1 + R_2 \longrightarrow \emptyset$$
$$S_2 + R_2 \longrightarrow S^+$$
$$S_2 + R_1 \longrightarrow \emptyset$$

4. When a predetermined frequency criterion for (a) correct responding and (b) the absence of incorrect responding have both been reached (typically ten successive errorless trials), move on to the next pair. Pairs should be dealt with in order from the easiest discrimination to the most difficult.

5. Each discrimination should also meet a criterion of generality, which can be tested by observations of the client's behavior in a variety of natural settings. Special transfer activities, in which discrimination is actually trained in natural settings, may also be required.

VICARIOUS CONDITIONING

Vicarious conditioning, in which modeled behavior is acquired by an observer, does not have to be seen from a cognitive point of view, since it is quite possible to describe it with reference only to observable events. But some of its characteristics implicate cognition as an important aspect of this learning process.

In the prototypical form of vicarious instrumental conditioning, a client observes a model performing a behavior and being reinforced for it, and as a result of the observation, the client's tendency to perform the same response is also increased. Modeled behaviors need not be actually reinforced in the presence of the observer. The model, if possessing characteristics such as authority and status, is presumed to gain reinforcement for whatever behaviors are modeled. So, given an appropriate model, no observed reinforcement is necessary.

Vicarious conditioning occurs most readily if the observer has some ability to use language already. Consequently, the earliest language forms are probably acquired by some other process, such as classical conditioning, as suggested earlier. Vicarious conditioning is also easier if the observer has been previously reinforced for matching the model's behavior. Therefore, in clinical applications, it is wise to begin a vicarious procedure with direct reinforcement for matching responses.

It is important not to confuse vicarious conditioning with imitation. Imitation suggests an exact copying of complex behaviors. In vicarious conditioning, the observer abstracts a general principle of behavior from the observation which he applies in similar situations generatively. Rule-learning occurs because the observer sees the response as an example from a broad category of responses and the circumstances (discriminative stimulus) as an example of a broad category of stimuli. This means that an observer seeing a model performing a particular response (R_1) in a particular context (S_1) acquires a tendency to perform the same response *and others of the same category* ($R_{1,2,\ldots,N} = R_A$) under the same circumstances *and other circumstances of the same category* ($S_{1,2,\ldots N}, = S_A$). The S_A and R_A symbols stand for categories of stimuli and responses. Thus, vicarious instrumental conditioning is shown by

$$S_A + R_A \longrightarrow S^{(+)}$$

where R_A = responses of type A, exemplified by $R_{1,2,\ldots,N}$, and S_A = stimuli of type A, exemplified by $S_{1,2,\ldots,N}$. The parentheses around the plus sign allow for inferred reinforcement. For example, the pluralization rules may be learned by observation of

$$S_A + R_A \longrightarrow S^{(+)}$$
$$S_B + R_B \longrightarrow S^{(+)}$$
$$S_C + R_C \longrightarrow S^{(+)}$$

where S_A = words ending in voiced sounds, S_B = words ending in unvoiced sounds, S_C = words ending in sibilants, R_A = /–z/, R_B = /–s/, and R_C = /–əz/.

The order of development in which these and similar rules are acquired—(1) specific lexical items, (2) abstraction of the rule and overgeneralization of it, producing errors, such as "I got two feets," and (3) refinement through discrimination between regular and irregular forms—is consistent with the idea that processes such as vicarious conditioning are responsible for it. The first few observations tie the rule to specific lexical items. Then the rule is abstracted and applied to all forms. Finally, the irregular exceptions are learned.

The categorical nature of vicarious conditioning allows for a description of the syntactic relations between words, and the cognitive structural relations to which they correspond. For example, in *John hit Mary, John* is a stimulus, S_1, but is also an example of the category of nouns (S_A). Similarly, *hit* is an example of the category of verbs. The cognitive events these words refer to, the idea of John and the idea of hitting, are also examples of categories of ideas, such as agents and actions. The position of the word *John* in front of the word *hit* may be considered a feature of the stimulus. The stimulus *John* (S_1) is made up of a number of features, one of which is its position in front of *hit*. Thus, a few sentences in which the noun precedes the verb are sufficient for the child to learn that this structure can be used to represent the agent-action relation. This more general rule is then abstracted and used generatively in productions of other sentences of the same structure. The main thing to realize is that the word order of a sentence is a legitimate stimulus and that the agent-action relation is a legitimate cognitive event.

The following procedure is useful in applying vicarious conditioning to the clinical instruction of language performance.

1. Identify the forms that are developmentally delayed and are desirable to teach, considering the child's present language performance, his needs which language might serve, normal developmental sequence, ease of training, and so on.

2. For each form, determine the appropriateness of vicarious conditioning at this stage in the child's acquisition of the form. I believe the best way to do this is with the very general three-step sequence already described: (1) specific lexical items, (2) rule abstraction and overgeneralization, and (3) refinement via discrimination. Clients who have not yet developed any specific lexical items containing the form are not ready to attempt rule abstraction. At the latter end of the sequence, clients who are making overgeneralization errors have already abstracted the rule. They may need discrimination training, but not vicarious conditioning. Only those clients who are in stage one in the development of the form should be scheduled for vicarious conditioning of that form.

3. Select a model. Models should have higher status than the client, typically by virtue of age, be competent speakers of the language, and yet be someone with whom the client can identify. Aides, students-in-training, and parents all fulfill these criteria.

4. Train the model. The object of vicarious conditioning is to show the client that the use of a certain form successfully communicates intention. The model must use the form while the client is attending, and it should be evident to the child that the model's intention was communicated. The clinician serves as a listener and reactor. It is not desirable to put on a little play for the client, with scripted parts and phony dialogue. Instead, explain the purpose of each session to the model, plan a well-structured series of interactions with a variety of interesting objects and activities, and then let in-

teractions between clinician and model occur as naturally as possible. In other words, establish general topics, then ad lib. A somewhat slower pace and stronger emphasis of the modeled form is probably helpful. The child can and should be part of the activity.

5. Train the child to match the model's behavior for a variety of (1) nonlangauge, then (2) language behaviors in the client's repertoire.
6. Carry out the procedure, reinforcing any of the client's behavior that matches the model's language behavior, not just the form in question.
7. Gradually restrict reinforcement to those responses that match the target form.
8. Assess performance for frequency and generality.
9. Introduce other forms.
10. Transfer the behavior to new settings. If generality criteria have been met, this should happen automatically. If not, additional modeling in extraclinical settings may be required, but I believe it is a tactical mistake to provide tangible reinforcement for a client's matching responses in extraclinical settings. The goal is self-reinforcement in extraclinical settings, and tangible reinforcers do not help to achieve it.

SELECTED REFERENCES

Bandura, A. *Principles of Behavior Modification*. New York: Holt, Rinehart, and Winston, Inc., 1969.

Bloom, L., and Lahey, M. *Language Development and Language Disorders*. New York: John Wiley and Sons, 1978.

Hilgard, E. and Marquis, D. (Eds.). *Conditioning and Learning*. New York: Appleton-Century-Crofts, Inc., 1961.

Starkweather, C. *Speech and Language: Principles and Processes of Behavior Change*. Englewood Cliffs, N.J.: Prentice-Hall, Inc., 1982.

CHAPTER FIVE

TECHNIQUES OF THERAPY BASED ON PRINCIPLES OF COUNSELING AND SELF-MANAGEMENT

Method of Deborah R. Klevans

I generally view my role in the therapeutic process as that of a consultant to the client who is seeking to remediate a communication disorder. My tasks are to enable the client to learn skills needed to establish more effective communication strategies, transfer new behaviors from treatment sessions to the natural environment, and maintain them over time.

The counseling process, which has been defined as the development of an effective interpersonal relationship, can contribute to these goals by establishing a structure within which change can take place. In the context of a positive relationship, the initial motivation to begin treatment can be sustained or increased, a model of effective interaction that promotes mutual respect and cooperation can be experienced, and support and skill training that enables the client to participate in planning and implementing behavior change and initiate self-management can be provided.

The skills used in counseling individuals with communication disorders and their families are the same as those used in a wide variety of effective interpersonal relationships, both formalized ones between a professional helper and the person seeking assistance, and those characterized by more mutuality and less formal role differentiation, such as those between peers or family members. In this broad sense, I use counseling with all clients throughout the course of treatment. However, the extent to which I use the counseling process as a central focus, particularly during the initial stages of treatment, varies considerably from client to client.

I have not found it fruitful to employ counseling as a primary strategy with clients whose intellectual, social-emotional, or language abilities are significantly impaired or markedly immature. Conversely, it is unnecessary to spend significant amounts of time counseling highly motivated clients with appropriate, realistic goals for improving their communication, who are committed to doing the work required.

Schultz and Carpenter (1973) have presented a useful perspective for differentiating between clients likely to benefit from systematic counseling and those ready to move immediately to the direct action phase of treatment or to dismissal. They suggest that if the client and clinician are in disagreement, or if either is uncertain about the desirability, possibility, or profitability of behavior change, then counseling is needed to seek an agreed-upon course of action.

While any counseling interaction is a complex interweaving of many elements that cannot be programmed in advance, a developmental model of helping, similar to one described by Gerard Egan (1975), is useful as a framework for organizing the counseling process. It consists of a preparation phase and three developmental stages, which trace the consideration of an issue from exploration to objective understanding to action or resolution. Often the process is repeated as additional issues arise during the course of treatment. (The purpose of each stage is noted in Table 1.)

PREPARATION PHASE

Naive clients may need to be prepared to participate as partners. There are several strategies I employ to this end. I sit directly across from the client, preferably without a table or desk between us, so that we can maintain eye contact and I can observe the client's nonverbal body language. I explain what is likely to occur during the treatment process and what I hope will be accomplished during this particular meeting. ("I'd like to understand what it's like for you to have this difficulty and what you hope to gain from treatment.") I also attempt to clarify and reach agreement regarding our roles (as active participant and facilitator), rights (to question, disagree, maintain confidentiality), and obligations (honesty, consideration, cooperation).

TABLE 1 Stages of a Developmental Counseling Model

Stage	*Purpose*
Preparation phase	Prepare client to participate actively in treatment process
Stage I. Exploration	Client and clinician develop mutual understanding of client's perspective
Stage II. Understanding	Client develops a relatively objective understanding of situation and alternatives for action
Stage III. Action	Client and clinician agree upon and implement action plan to modify client's behavior and develop skills needed to become self-manager

This sets the tone of our relationship as one in which the client is made as fully aware as possible of the reasons for undertaking a given activity rather than being the passive recipient of treatment.

I attempt to use language that is free of technical jargon and is easily understood by the client, and to speak slowly enough to allow for spontaneous questions or comments. In summary, I prefer an informal style that is as role-free as possible without denying the fact that as a professional I presumably bring skills to our interaction which the client has not mastered.

STAGE I—EXPLORING THE PROBLEM

The purpose of this stage is to enable a client to consider his communication difficulties from his own perspective as a basis for determining a course of action for dealing with them. My task is to provide an environment that encourages the client to explore concerns in concrete terms and to be understood. This is done in a manner which the client perceives as respectful, nonjudgmental, and honest.

Encouragers

In order to keep the focus on the client and promote his self-exploration, I use nonverbal encouragers such as affirmative head nods and responsive facial expressions and hand gestures. I also add occasional verbal encouragers such as "um-hmm," "Oh?" and "Go on." I avoid switching topics at this stage, letting the client take the lead.

Interchangeable Empathic Responses

To help the client move forward in focusing on critical issues, I communicate and verify my understanding by restating, in my own words, the essence of the ideas and feelings he has expressed. Such responses serve two purposes. First, they provide for a check on my basic comprehension of the intended message, particularly if the client's communication is not readily intelligible. Second, my concise review, presented with some tentativeness, allows the client to confirm or deny the accuracy of my perception. At this stage in our interaction, I usually limit my reflections to restatements of the explicit messages stated, avoiding interpretation or embellishment. ("Sounds like you were discouraged that the salesperson looked away when you spoke.")

Questions

If I become confused, have difficulty following the client's train of thought, or decide the client is too vague or has begun to ramble, I may ask some questions, preferably open-ended ones (such as "What exactly does your sister do which makes you think she gets impatient when you talk?"). Well-formed questions can help to clarify or refocus the narrative and encourage specificity and concreteness. Unless an issue eventually is discussed in operational terms, talk is unlikely to lead to increased understanding or action.

Self-Involving Feedback

Reinforcing comments are often productive at this point. ("I find it helpful when you share your experiences in this way.") If the client is reticent or seems unwilling to discuss a problem openly, I try to provide both support and gentle pressure by communicating my reaction openly. ("You seem to be having difficulty talking about this. I've been wondering if there is some way I can help you feel freer to express yourself.")

Summarization

When a topic has been adequately considered, I sometimes provide closure and a transition by summarizing what has been discussed. It may consist of a single thought ("From what you've said thus far, your stuttering has affected all of your relationships"), some conflicts or contradictions ("To sum up then, you're very anxious to regain your voice, but don't want to spend a lot of time and money for treatment"), or a series of thoughts ("If we were to list all of the positive attributes you bring to therapy they would include...").

If the client and I have worked well together up to this point, we will conclude the exploration stage of the counseling process with an awareness that we have a mutually shared perception of the client's communication problem as experienced by the client, and some appreciation of the strengths and resources the client brings to the treatment process.

STAGE II—GAINING OBJECTIVE UNDERSTANDING

The purpose of the second stage is for the client to build upon the information gathered previously in order to develop a more complete and objective understanding of his situation. The goal is to use this broadened perspective to make an informed decision about what, if any, further action to take. The self-understanding gained through this process often leads to enhanced motivation to follow through on an action plan as well.

While I continue to employ all of the communicative responses, I add my own perceptions and provide relevant information as needed. In order not to overwhelm the client, it is important to provide a supportive relationship and to proceed cautiously and tentatively in using the potentially more potent responses described in the following sections.

Additive Empathic Responses

I continue to reflect the ideas and feelings expressed by the client, but begin to add depth by including indications of what the client's communication seems to imply as well as what was expressed directly. This differs from analysis or diagnosis in that I don't suggest a label or use theoretical constructs. If accurate and well-timed, these higher level empathic responses have the effect of enabling the client to understand the situation more completely. ("Putting so much effort into speaking and yet being misunderstood really annoys you. I sense that it makes you feel sorry for yourself at times, too.")

Self-Disclosure

Occasionally I find it helpful to share personal information or an experience of my own with the client. Indicating that I, too, am struggling to balance the demands of a job and a family, or that my experience in relearning to ride a bike after being in an accident has some parallels with the risk taking he is now contemplating, can enhance the client's self-understanding and strengthen our relationship by emphasizing our commonalities. This is constructive as long as I do not use it as a means of dealing with my own needs or deflecting the client from dealing with his concerns. It is also useful only to the extent that my experiences are similar enough to have some direct application.

Confrontation

A more potent form of sharing my views is to indicate discrepancies, distortions, or self-deceptions that have become apparent to me in the course of the client's self-exploration. Realizing that it is often difficult for someone to be confronted, I present these remarks tentatively and in the context of my caring for the client. This can only be done if and when I sense that our relationship is sufficiently strong to withstand the discomfort that is likely to follow. It is important to follow a confronting remark by attending to both the verbal and nonverbal responses of the client and by conveying empathic understanding of the feelings that have been engendered. ("It's painful for you to face these conflicts in yourself.")

Confrontation may be used to focus on a number of factors that have the potential to interfere with the development of a constructive and practical action plan. For example, discrepancies between stated intentions and behavior can be highlighted. ("You've mentioned how determined you are to improve your speech, yet this is the third session for which you've been late.") Confrontation can also be appropriate in resolving issues that affect the immediate relationship between clinician and client if, for example, I become so annoyed by the client's habitual lateness that it affects my ability to respond positively. ("I have become so irritated by your lateness that it's difficult for me to respond to you with care and understanding. I think it's important for us to resolve this.")

Presenting Alternative Interpretations

Often clients come for treatment with preconceptions or inaccurate information, which is likely to interfere with appropriate decision-making and constructive change. During this stage of the counseling process I may find it helpful to provide input that gives the client an opportunity to consider an issue from new perspectives. These alternative interpretations can be presented in the form of statements for consideration ("Is it possible that your friend looks away when you talk not because he's impatient, but because he's not sure how to respond?"), shared knowledge ("These are some of the things we do know about the way in which language develops"), or by encouraging the client to consider alternative interpretations ("What are some other reasons your mother may have started crying?").

Summarizing

I continue to use summarizing statements as I did earlier. They are useful in this stage, not only as a means of focusing and reviewing an extended discussion, but also as a means of drawing together relevant themes and leading the client to a consideration of an appropriate course of action.

The second stage of counseling is successfully concluded if the client is able to be a full participant in reaching decisions regarding future actions that represent his own self-interests and are based on a reasonably objective understanding of the problem and the resources available to cope with it. Another consideration is whether the costs of implementing an action plan are worthwhile in relation to the value that the anticipated behavior change will have.

If the client and I do not agree that participation in a treatment program that I can provide is needed, possible, and/or worthwhile, then it follows that treatment should be terminated or that help be sought elsewhere. If, on the other hand, we agree that working together to implement a treatment program is desirable, we are ready to move to the third, or action, stage of the clinical relationship.

STAGE III—IMPLEMENTING ACTION

The client's goals in this stage are to achieve mastery of two separate but related sets of tasks. The first set involves the establishment of improved communicative ability, the goal to which most of the books in this series are addressed. The second is to become an effective self-manager who is able to transfer and maintain newly acquired communication skills in everyday activities.

Although research data concerning the effectiveness of particular self-management strategies are limited, Frederick Kanfer, in summarizing much of the available information, notes that prior to implementing a self-management program it is important to ensure that the client is motivated to change, is ready to accept major responsibility for implementing change, and is working with someone with whom a positive relationship has been developed.

The first task in assisting a client to develop and use self-management strategies is to foster the acquisition of needed skills not already learned. Skills specific to behavior change and self-management will be considered individually in the next section. The more general abilities involved, such as decision-making and goal-setting, are beyond the scope of this chapter.

I find it effective to structure the overall treatment program so that self-management procedures are an integral component of treatment from the start. They can be incorporated into most treatment approaches by encouraging the client to be an active partner in deciding among available and appropriate treatment options, planning sessions, monitoring and assessing performance, and determining and administering appropriate reinforcements.

Once these skills are established, it is through the use of homework assignments that have been planned, rehearsed, and later evaluated that the client assumes increasingly greater responsibility for changing old patterns. By carefully monitoring these early efforts, I can begin to shape and reinforce the client's attempts at self-management long before he is completely on his own.

SELF-MANAGEMENT SKILLS

Self-Assessment

The client must learn to identify, analyze, and record target behaviors. Both self-monitoring and self-evaluation are involved in these tasks. The client begins to learn these skills by sharing the assessment and evaluation tasks with me during treatment sessions. After discussing the importance of accurate record-keeping in determining progress, I demonstrate my procedure for keeping data. It usually involves use of frequency counts for recording discrete behaviors such as correct phoneme production, time-sampling or time-interval measures for continuous behaviors such as reading aloud at a given rate, and rating scales for more qualitative or subjective measures.

The client practices attending to, identifying, and recording specified behaviors and comparing his scores with mine. Once we reach reasonable interrater reliability, we consider methods for gathering similar data in other settings. Methods that are both practical and unobstrusive are preferred. A wrist-worn or hand-held counter is useful for making frequency counts. Infrequently occurring behaviors can be recorded by transferring small objects such as pennies or toothpicks from one pocket to another. A wristwatch with a second hand or a stopwatch can be used for time-interval recording.

It is important to rehearse the exact procedures to be used with the client, using the same paraphernalia he will be using. Role-playing, or practicing in as life-like a situation as possible, is desirable. The client's first attempts at self-monitoring should be done in as stress-free and supportive an environment as possible. They should be reviewed in detail at the next treatment session to determine whether any modifications in the agreed-upon procedures are needed. If the behavior to be monitored is a complex one, it is helpful, where feasible, if the client tape-records the interaction being monitored, and then compares the on-the-spot scoring with our joint efforts at monitoring from the tape, as we listen to it together later on.

Establishing Effective Consequences

I usually suggest the use of behavior modification strategies in designing a self-management program. Therefore, I ask the client to generate a list of positive consequences to self-administer following the successful completion of a task, and help him become adept at doing so appropriately. When I explain the need for self-administered awards, some adult clients are resistant to what they deem to be a childish approach. However, if a rationale is given and a sense of humor and some creativity employed, most clients enjoy the procedure.

When compiling a list of reinforcers, it is imperative that the client be the final judge of the list. It must, of course, consist of items that are rewarding to the client, not necessarily to the clinician. The list should be as varied as possible. It could include material rewards (a magazine, a cup of coffee, cosmetics, money), activities (TV watching, reading, jogging, working on a hobby), and verbal or symbolic acts (making positive self-statements, adding a data point or a star to a progress graph). The importance of providing reinforcement as soon as possible following the completion of the target behavior should be emphasized. As is true for self-monitoring, it is important for most clients to administer self-reinforcements during treatment sessions first, and then practice doing so in other settings under supervision, if possible, before trying to take over their own reinforcement schedules.

Arranging a Supportive Environment

Frequently, clients who are not successful in carrying out agreed-upon self-management procedures blame their lack of success on external factors. ("I kept being interrupted. I didn't have money to use the pay phone. No one was around to talk with.") When this happens, it is helpful to discuss with the client what barriers are likely to prevent the completion of a particular assignment. Together, we consider ways to reduce or eliminate barriers. For example, we determine where to work without interruption, arrange to obtain change for the telephone ahead of time, make plans to meet a particular person with whom to talk.

We also consider ways to use external factors to increase the possibility of success. I might encourage the client to tell others of his plans and to request that they inquire about his progress. We might discuss the least expensive place to purchase needed equipment. We might consider when disruptive family members are least likely to be around before working out a schedule for practicing reading aloud.

The more specifically and clearly self-management procedures are defined, the more likely they are to be implemented. "Why don't you practice as much as you can this week" is a common suggestion, usually doomed to failure.

Developing Contracts

The procedures described thus far lend themselves readily to the development of contracts for out-of-clinic assignments. Contracts provide a structure for implementing self-management techniques in a practical way. Although they are most often written in behavioral terms, individuals who dislike a highly structured approach may choose instead to write homework assignments in the form of a series of directions.

I usually lay the foundation for this phase of self-management by asking the client to assist in writing plans for treatment sessions in which communication skills are being established. Once capable of describing objectives, procedures, and reinforcement schedules, the client is ready to begin planning homework contracts. Of course, clients vary considerably in the extent to which they are able to carry out these tasks independently. Whatever the amount of help required in writing the contracts, they usually include the components indicated in the example presented below:

> I will say hello (behavior objective) to between five and ten strangers (measured in terms of frequency counts) while walking home via Main Street (environmental variable contributing to likelihood of success). I will keep track of each greeting by using my hand counter (means for measuring). As soon as I have completed the minimum number of greetings (5) I may go directly home and watch the news on TV (positive consequence).

An optional addition may be included if an aversive consequence seems desirable in the event the task is not completed:

> If I haven't completed the minimum number of greetings by the time I arrive home, I will walk on to the neighborhood shopping center and continue walking around there until I complete my goal. Then I will go home.

Home assignments in any form are more likely to be done if they are perceived as consisting of manageable tasks, similar to ones that the client has successfully practiced in treatment sessions, which take into account time and environmental limitations as well as the client's psychological readiness for risk-taking.

RETURNING TO THE BEGINNING

I began this chapter with the notion that a developmental-counseling model is circular, not linear. Experienced clinicians are well aware that, in the course of treatment, it is almost inevitable that clients will have problems that may interfere with their ability to complete even the most carefully considered plan. If difficulties cannot be surmounted by modifying the program or providing additional information, it may be that such factors as fear, resistance to change, or decreasing motivation may be operating. If so, it is often useful to return, however briefly, to Stage I of the counseling process and encourage the client to explore the problem more fully. The resulting self-understanding is likely to lead to a renewed commitment to resuming the original, or a revised, action plan. I have found that implementing the counseling process during the later stages of treatment is often helpful even for clients for whom counseling was not needed initially.

SELECTED REFERENCES

Egan, G. *The Skilled Helper*. Monterey, California: Brooks/Cole Publishing Company, 1975.

Goldstein, A., and Kanfer, F. (Eds.). *Maximizing Treatment Gains: Transfer Enhancement in Psychotherapy*. New York: Academic Press, 1979.

Kanfer, F., and Goldstein, A. (Eds.). *Helping People Change: A Textbook of Methods (2nd Edition)*. New York: Pergamon Press, 1980.

Klevans, D., Volz, H., and Friedman, R. A comparison of experiential and observational approaches for enhancing the interpersonal communication skills of speech-langauge pathology students. *Journal of Speech and Hearing Disorders*, 1981, 46:208-212.

Schultz, M., and Carpenter, M. The bases of speech pathology and audiology: Selecting a therapy model. *Journal of Speech and Hearing Disorders*, 1973, 38:395-404

CHAPTER SIX

TECHNIQUES OF THERAPY BASED ON PRINCIPLES OF PSYCHOTHERAPY

Method of Clyde L. Rousey

At least 95 percent of my patients with articulation and voice disorders are treated by psychoanalytically oriented psychotherapy. As a way of understanding the use of psychotherapy as well as just what psychotherapy is, it is useful to note that at most universities in the 1950s speech problems were viewed primarily from an organic perspective. Thus the more recent shift to a predominantly psychological viewpoint represented a rather radical change. I think it safe to say that most of my colleagues in speech pathology continue to feel most comfortable in using some variant of the organic model or some variant of learning theory in both their diagnosis and treatment of speech disorders.

PROBLEMS WITH THE CONVENTIONAL ORIENTATION

After years of attempts to treat speech disorders by use of "ear training," "moto-kinesthetic methods," or some form of reward for correct production of sound, it became painfully aware to me that while a "cure" of a sound substitution was easily accomplished in my office, the harsh reality was that it rarely carried over outside. It also became clear from association with colleagues who later embraced operant procedures that the same issue reared its head again under the designation of a lack of generalization. I also was troubled by popular explanations of why some sounds were easier to change in my office, e.g., by ear training, than others. This was especially so since studies regarding sound discrimination ability of speech-defective children were and continue to be inconclusive at best. Also, I knew that what were being called discrimination problems by speech pathologists were not what audiologists meant by that term. Thus, the possibility had to be entertained that the whole issue of sound discrimination as a factor in articulation was a red herring. McDonald's observation years ago that regardless of the articulation error, one could find a place where it was produced correctly, also would argue against any articulation problem resulting from an innate discrimination problem. The explanation of some sounds being easier to change because they were more visible or easier to produce, while interesting as a hypothetical construct and perhaps satisfying to a parent, simply did not have internal consistency. That is, if this hypothesis were correct, then no one should have trouble producing, for example, a "p" sound and everyone should have trouble producing, for example, a "g" sound. That such a verity does not exist goes without question. It is interesting that the longer one labors in a field of study, the more one sees an old idea coming around for another go with a new generation of students. This is nowhere better demonstrated than by the current focus on distinctive features as a way of understanding misarticulations. The same problems arose for me in this formulation as I already have detailed. Finally, I was troubled by the neurologic model for explaining articulation problems. Admittedly, in cases where there was clear damage to various parts of the brain, it was easy to assume a cause-and-effect relationship. However, even in these instances, observation of undeniably neurologically impaired patients clearly demonstrated that their dysarthrias were variable. The real difficulty appeared when I tried to apply this conceptual framework to the vast majority of children and adults with disturbed articulation where no independent evidence of neurologic pathology existed.

Further, although I had read and believed Templin's data and told many a parent that it was normal not to say the voiceless *th* or voiced *th* at age three, the actual fact I discovered, both as a parent and observer, was that this assumption was not tenable for all children. When I went back to reread Templin, I discovered that she clearly did not say that any one sound totally develops at a specific age. Her data were further substantiated in research by Hall and Healy. Thus, the developmental notions of speech acquisition did not explain the observable facts and consequently posed too many complications for clinical use.

The final straw that made me believe there must be a better conceptualization of articulation and voice problems occurred when I had the opportunity to assess the speech of psychiatric patients at The Menninger Foundation. It very quickly became apparent that at least 90 percent of these patients—whether children or adults—had varying articulation and voice problems. Such a high prevalence had to be explained. Worse yet was the realization that many of them had had speech therapy in schools and clinics and had been considered cured. I discovered that my observations about speech abilities of patients in this sample of our population were not the result of any bias or blind spot peculiar to me. Indeed, numerous other studies conducted around the United States by clinicians and researchers were reporting the same phenomenon. Finally, when I followed these patients through their psychiatric treatment, I discovered that in successful psychotherapy the speech problem went away, whereas in treatment failures the speech difficulty remained. The inescapable fact appeared to be that good psychotherapists were also, unbeknowst to themselves, good speech therapists.

MY WORK ON THE PROBLEMS

With these troublesome issues needing reconciliation, I was fortunate to become involved in a post-doctoral experience at The Menninger Foundation. This institution has a predominant psychoanalytic orientation. While this way of viewing psychologic development is not as popular as it once was, it still remains the most comprehensive psychologic position for both clinical practice and research that has been developed, for it takes into account both cognitive and affective development. Most of our theories in speech pathology emphasize solely the cognitive part of mental functioning. Such an emphasis reflects a belief that to do so is to be rational and, inferentially, scientific. It also has occurred because most of our training institutions in speech pathology have neither the staff nor the inclination to view the contributions of both cognition and affect as they are reflected through speech.

A further problem has been our professional heritage which, while contributing to our growth, has focused on neurological or learning disturbances as causative factors. It was thus small wonder that psychotherapy as a treatment of choice for speech disorders attracted both minimal and negative attention, since it was not within the background realm of my professors (neurologists, otolaryngologists, educators, or cognitively oriented academicians). Further, as a young therapist I was taught that while there may be some secondary emotional reactions to a speech disorder, these will go away if I treat the speech problem. The human and natural rivalry between disciplines further contributes to the problem by making it difficult to conceive of anyone from "another field" really understanding and being able to contribute to our profession. When these limitations are combined with the popularized negative image of psychoanalysis, I can understand why "responsible clinicians" would eschew this approach.

DEVELOPMENT OF A PSYCHOLOGICAL EXPLANATION

Elsewhere, I have written extensively on a theoretical position that bridges the gap between our knowledge of speech production and psychological growth as viewed from a psychoanalytic viewpoint. In such a brief chapter as this, repetition of this material is not only impractical, but impossible. However, a broad outline of the critical assumptions is necessary to see how psychotherapy is applicable to speech disorders.

If the reader will recall Irwin's early studies of sound development, they showed that by one year of age all the various vowels and consonants had been uttered. This painstaking research, conducted in the days before tape recording was universal, represents an enormous and dedicated effort as well as living proof of the importance of basic research. In broad terms, Irwin and his students discovered that vowels seem to be the predominant sound uttered in the first 6 months of life, whereas consonants appear en masse the last 6 months of the first year. Most surely, I reasoned, this phenomenon demonstrated that sound production was independent of spoken language in the vast majority of persons. The exceptions to this (e.g., the person who has a congenital and profound hearing loss) represent a small but, of course, not unimportnat part of our population. Consequently, the fact that children had trouble using sounds in words could not be explained by such simple reasons as (1) a motor difficulty (for they had already said them), (2) an auditory perceptual problem (they had already said and heard them), or (3) a cognitive skill (they had already produced them).

Psychological Meaning of Vowels

Viewed from this context, the use and misuse of sounds clearly required another explanation. When one understands psychological development from a psychoanalytic view, some new and interesting possibilities emerge. For example, it is generally accepted that infants in their first 6 months have two primary urges, which they both express and seek to have gratified. Specifically, they want to feel loved and nurtured, and will express their anger and frustration over being hungry or uncomfortable. The intensity of these issues lessens only when infants can exert some control and realize that they are separate individuals from their parents. This separation and individuation process has been described in detail by Mahler and her colleagues. Given our knowledge regarding sound development and what Mahler has termed the psychological birth of the human infant, it seemed plausible to hypothesize that vowels may well be a primary way of communicating these predictable urges of the infant. This is further illustrated by a mother's use of sound in responding to her child's needs. I also assumed that difficulties with vowels in later life reflected early and continuing problems in expression of basic drives or urges (aggression and sexuality, creativity and caring).

Psychological Meaning of Consonants

During the second 6 months of life, children psychologically continue their separation and individuation from their parents. They become increasingly aware of the need for relationships and their increasingly complex development in both affect and cognition allows them to begin controlling their relationships with others. Because specific adjustments and controls are needed to produce consonants, and consonants also appear largely in the second 6 months of life, it seemed reasonable to hypothesize that the development of consonants may be closely related to infants' awareness of their parents, and their developing feelings vis-à-vis these important persons. An alternative explanation might be offered by my neurologically oriented colleagues that central nervous system (CNS) maturation was responsible for the increased motor skills involved in making consonants. For this explanation to wash clean, it would be necessary to have a more discrete understanding of CNS development than we presently have. The explanation I chose (i.e., the emerging emotional relationships) is at this point easier to demonstrate. For, if it is correct, these disruptions or disturbances in these relationships should manifest themselves later in sound-making difficulties. In other words, I reasoned that the anlage of consonant difficulties occurring because of parental relationship problems were laid down in the second half of the first year of life and, like a radioactive tracer, appeared again in later years in response to emotional conflict at home or elsewhere.

In my assumptions, the fact that both consonants and vowels were made perfectly at one time or the other during the first year of life allowed for understanding problems in their correct use at a later date as a symptom of emotional development gone awry. A corollary of this position would be that persons having no unusual emotional conflicts, and in whom emotional development is "normal," would show no later errors in their speech. Such an explanatory position finally allowed an understanding of why some children had no speech problems while others had many. I also indicated that there is no such thing as a minor speech problem (i.e., only one error as opposed to two or more). Whenever one speech error is present, a problem in emotional growth and development has occurred. I knew such a position would complicate the practicing clinician's professional life in terms of choosing which child's speech problems needed attention. On the other hand, if true, it had enormous implications for what is being taught in our graduate schools. In my other writings, I have both explicated as well as provided clinical research to develop and test the plausibility of these notions.

Importance of Diagnosis Before Psychotherapy

What I am alluding to is the primary need for a diagnosis before beginning psychotherapy. It has become increasingly popular in some circles to begin psychotherapy without such a diagnosis. Part of this reaction is traceable to an attempt to get away from what some therapists feel is the evil "medical model." In so doing, they have often thrown the baby out with the bath water. (There are also other social, professional, and political issues involved that deserve more attention than possible in this context.)

At any rate, by using the theoretical schema I have proposed, it is possible to come to a diagnostic understanding of such important areas of mental status as early child/parent relationships, mastery of such milestones of psychological development as independence, sharing, development of sexual identity, degree of depression and inhibition, and so on. For example, understanding the interdependence between speech development and psychological development becomes important for using psychotherapy as a modality of treatment. For, knowing that a substitution of *f* for the voiceless *th* was related to a psychological absence of paternal figures, makes for a better understanding of either the play or talking with the patient with a speech problem. Further, our increasing knowledge of the psychological contribution of fathers to their childrens' emotional growth and development would make us understand troubles such children are experiencing as having different roots than, for example, what is seen in children rejected by their mothers.

Alongside the diagnostic picture drawn from the speech data, I find it important to consider the results of psychologic testing, social casework interviews, psychiatric observations, and consultations by medical specialists such as a neurologist. In general, along with my colleagues in psychology and psychiatry, I have found failure in psychotherapy to be (1) a primary function of poor or incomplete diagnosis and (2) caused by complications resulting from a poorly trained therapist. Since most of my colleagues have no formal training in psychotherapy, use of this modality will probably fail. As in clinical psychology, such a development must also probably await the development of post-doctoral programs that are integrated with psychology, psychiatry, and social work.

JUST WHAT IS PSYCHOTHERAPY?

In talking with my colleagues in speech pathology about psychotherapy, I find there is a reluctance to consider it, not ony because of the factors mentioned but also because they do not understand psychoanalysis and are confused as to just what psychotherapy is. This problem, in part, reflects the frequent proclivity for therapists of any persuasion to call what they do "psychotherapy." This occurs for political, economic, and professional reasons. The estimated 200 treatment approaches labelled as "psychotherapy" documents this point. Further, the meteoric rise and fall of the various self-help programs demonstrates their faddish character and inadequacies. My discussion of psychotherapy is based solely on psychoanalytic assumptions. (Various other approaches to psychotherapy are available in the psychologic and psychiatric literature.) Whenever I talk to groups, I find that when psychoanalysis is mentioned, the usual reaction is that it has something to do with sex and "besides, it is outmoded and a dead theory." This response is due in part to my auditors never having read the complete works of Freud, as well as their failing to keep up with current developments in psychoanalytic literature. Reports of the death of psychoanalysis, to paraphrase a famous saying, are premature and exaggerated. Indeed, perusal of the professional literature and actions by psychologists interested in psychoanalysis will demonstrate quite the contrary.

In a contribution such as this, it is only possible to summarize some of the main things we do when we provide psychoanalytically oriented psychotherapy. To actually use this form of treatment requries extensive training and supervision.

Psychoanalytic psychotherapy is usually conceived of as supportive or expressive, or some combination of both. In general, supportive psychotherapy focuses the person's attention on here and now issues without asking him to consider unconscious determinants. In contrast, expressive psychotherapy involves work on unconscious determinants as they are manifested through various behavioral, affective, and cognitive acts. While dividing psychotherapy into such a dichotomy is often done for teaching purposes, it belies the fact that actual therapy for most persons emphasizes both elements to some degree.

Candidates for Psychotherapy

Generally speaking, a patient who is in conflict over relationships with other people is the best candidate. Since my conceptualization of speech problems involves parent-child conflict as an etiologic agent, speech-disordered individuals are prime candidates. Further, some capacity for communication is required. This can be done either through words (spoken or signed) or through play. The more severe the retardation, the less likely is psychotherapy to be used. Also, the greater the person's disturbance in thought organization and character pathology, the more complicated treatment becomes. Happily, character pathology is not a clinical issue in the preschool and elementary school-age child. Unfortunately, the degree of thought organization and reality testing is rarely considered unless the child is blatantly autistic or psychotic. Since most child therapists are reluctant to diagnose children as such, it is not given the proper attention. However, thought disorganization in the absence of organicity can be treated by psychotherapy.

IMPORTANT CONSIDERATIONS

Transference

I attempt in psychotherapy to allow children or adults to recreate in their relationships with me the same kind of relationships they had with their mothers and fathers. The responses and reactions they make are part of the process of transference. The heart of treatment is helping the patient understand these early relationships and how they are acted out in the present. In the case of an articulation or voice disorder resulting from psychologic factors, the task is to help the patient understand the conflict embodied in the speech symptomatology and how it interferes not only with communication, but also with emotional well-being. However, to understand the transference phenomenon fully requires knowledge on my part of my own feelings and early relationships with my parents. If I do not know this, the risk is high that I will infuse some of my own problems into my treatment. When this happens, a phenomenon termed countertransference is said to occur. However, if I am aware of how my patient's actions arouse feelings in me, and I use these feelings to help the patient understand his own problems, the phenomenon of countertransference can be useful. To overcome these potential treatment complications, most therapists have had a treatment experience of their own and have professional supervision of their psychotherapy throughout several complete cases. All good therapists continue to make use of collegial supervision throughout their career. Anyone who thinks he can practice psychotherapy solely as a result of reading this or other material is in for a disappointment. Worse yet, he will be doing a disservice to the patient.

Negative and Positive Feelings

Both these feelings are identifiable in the transference. It is preferable when the person I am treating cooperates. In conventional speech therapy, it is often easier for boys to correct their speech problems temporarily for their pretty therapist and for girls to do the same for their handsome male therapist. Such a response is termed a positive transference cure and occurs frequently in incomplete psychotherapy processes. Most of my early failures were in not recognizing that my patients also had negative and angry feelings about me, their speech, and their parents. Not recognizing meant, in my case, not treating. Thus, it was small wonder they reverted to their speech difficulties when they had finished their appointment and had to return to the conflicts with their parents which had precipated the problems.

Communication in Psychotherapy

Communicating in psychotherapy can be either through words or play. In many children I see who have speech problems or who are failing to begin talking, I must resort to play while using talk with their parents or relatives. Other than during the diagnostic part of my contact with the patient, I generally allow the patient to talk about what he wishes. By this method I know that important areas will surface during the course of our developing relationship. Understanding these areas within the context of psychoanalytic theory allows for both their conflicts and their needs. My understanding of the psychological meanings of their speech problems allows me to respond more quickly than if I had to wait for them to express their conflicts via the multiple meanings that are attached to words and language. This phenomenon is termed overdeterminism and is not addressed in current cognitive approaches to language disorders. Ultimately, this issue will become the Achilles heel for any schema that claims to understand or treat language production.

Rewards for Patients

Another important feature of psychotherapy involves providing no other gratification to the patient than the presence and understanding of the therapist. The practice of providing reinforcers (e.g., candy, toys) can play into the psychopathology of a patient. For example, it is not unheard of that a person with a *w* for *r* substitution will respond to various reinforcement schedules so long as a reward is given, but then revert to the old speech problem afterward. That this occurs reflects in part the conflict of such an individual over giving and receiving. Such persons usually have great skills initially in complying passively, but in the end defeat the best efforts of the therapist. Further, giving concrete rewards becomes tantamount to bribing or paying ransom. Society knows that while this has been often tried, the true motivation for lasting change must come from within a person.

Frequency of Psychotherapy

As a general rule, I provide psychotherapy two to three times a week. This frequency of contact encourages sufficient development of a transference for treatment to proceed. The brief contact most speech therapists have dilutes and inhibits any potential for development of transference. In addition, I schedule parent conferences in which what I do is essentially casework. Under no circumstances do I send home work to be done or have the parents "drill" their children. Focus with the parents, as with the child, is on both positive and negative psychological factors. As those who give psychotherapy know, children repeat the psychological difficulties of their parents. It may well be this issue which seems to produce similar speech difficulties in parents and their children and which, in the past, has been interpreted as "inherited" speech problems. In truth, no biological inheritance need have occurred. In a broad sense, there is some obvious pyschological inheritance operative.

Ending Treatment

Termination of psychotherapy for persons with speech problems comes when speech is improved and the conflicts expressed in the speech difficulty have been resolved. At that point, old speech difficulties may reappear briefly. I have noted, even in patients whose speech has improved, that given the proper amount of stress, their old speech problems will reappear. This phenomenon is understandable, not as a failure of treatment, but as a reflection that, under stress, all of us revert to the point of our greatest past weakness. This phenomenon is not peculiar to psychotherapy, for architects know a building will buckle at the weakest structural point. Incidentally, I have observed not only in myself, but also in others, the transient appearance of speech difficulties. Knowing myself and the meaning of these problems allows me to cope psychologically. Indeed, given the right circumstance, I am sure I could induce a transient speech problem in anyone.

In my experience, articulation and voice production are indescribably delicate expressions of mental stability. Treating disturbances in talking as symptomatic of emotional distress produces substantive and lasting changes. Diagnosis and treatment must consider both the cognitive and emotional sides of a person's life.

SELECTED REFERENCES

Blanck, G., and Blanck, R. *Ego Psychology: Theory and Practice*. New York; Columbia University Press, 1974.

Mahler, M., Pine, F., and Bergman, A. *The Psychological Birth of the Human Infant*. New York; Basic Books, Inc., 1975.

Rousey, C. *Psychiatric Assessment by Speech and Hearing Behavior*. Springfield, Illinois: Charles C. Thomas, 1974.

CHAPTER SEVEN

TREATMENT OF CHILDREN BASED ON PRINCIPLES OF PSYCHOTHERAPY

Method of Lois W. Douglass

Psychotherapy is a self-exploratory process. Its success is dependent upon an important but rarely discussed communication skill: the ability to transform amorphous thoughts and feelings into meaningful words. My interest in the psychotherapeutic process led me to believe that the development of this skill should be included in the therapy of children with speech disorders. The therapy I will describe is designed to do just that. Freedom of choice of activity in a play environment allows the child to explore his environment and make discoveries about himself as he relates to that environment.

Words, spoken by the child and the therapist, form the core of the therapy. These words are attached to the child's actions, thoughts, and feelings as he plays.* Now labeled, those actions, thoughts, and feelings achieve the permanence that allows the child to store his external and internal worlds in his memory, selectively and effectively. At a later date, he can draw on this important store of knowledge of himself and his environment to problem solve. He will have the ability to use speech as a coping tool.

Little direct attention is given to the sound and structure of speech and language. The child's articulation, syntax, grammar, vocabulary, vocal quality, and fluency change as he identifies with the speech and language of his therapist.

Therapy has been designed to promote the social growth (including development and/or refinement of communication skills) and the emotional growth of any child. It is very effective with children of normal intelligence whose speech and language are delayed and/or severely disordered. Young children who stutter also respond well. Positive changes in speech, language, and self-esteem have been seen in Downs syndrome children with whom I have worked.

Children with serious emotional problems should be referred to a psychiatrist, psychologist, or social worker who specializes in psychotherapy.

---

*For simplicity's sake, I will refer to the child as "he," the therapist as "she."

PREREQUISITES FOR SUCCESSFUL TREATMENT IN A PLAY ENVIRONMENT

Competency of the therapist. The competency of the therapist depends heavily upon: (1) knowledge of the psychosocial and physical development of the child, including the development of speech and language; (2) understanding of the dynamics of interpersonal relationships; and (3) an eagerness to know more about (1) and (2). The therapist's ability to listen to and talk to a child and/or his parents easily is also of utmost importance. How well she can do this may depend on her awareness of her own personal trouble spots. At times, my patients and their parents present problems that trigger within me memories surrounding unresolved problems. Therefore, when I feel discomfort over what I hear or observe, attending to the cause of my discomfort is important. I do not want to read into my client's or his parents' behavior something that belongs to me, not them.

Ability of parent and child to separate. In many cases, parents and their child with disordered speech are bound together by the speech disorder. Normally, a child seriously begins to reach out to explore the world beyond his parents when he begins to develop speech and language. At this time, the bond between the child and his parents loosens in order that the child may become an individual. This process is known as separation-individuation. A speech disorder tends to tighten the parent-child bond. The child reaches out to his parents for comfort and protection when his communication skills fail him. In turn, parents reach out to comfort and protect their child. As a result the normal, important, elastic bonding becomes more of a bondage.

The need for privacy in therapy demands separation of the parents and their child. It is my task to make the separation possible without creating a sense of loss in either parent or child—a difficult task I keep in mind throughout therapy. I also consider the fact that the child's speech disorder is a bonding agent in my relationship with the child. The ease with which my patient moves back to his parents is a prime concern of therapy. *My goal is not separation of parent and child, but a healthy bonding between them*

Suitable Environment. The therapeutic environment should be one in which the child has freedom to move and freedom to choose from a broad variety of activities. I store all toys and games in cupboards, which are closed on the child's entry into the room. This makes certain that his choices are his, rather than mine or the child who came before him. I provide individual lockers for each of my patients, so that they can store "valuables" or toys they wish to use, as if they were their own private property.

PLAY DESCRIBED

Play begins as a free flow of physical and psychic energy experienced when one is in a state of well-being. This free flow of energy is not goal-oriented and so moves in any direction that internal needs and environmental opportunities will take it. The end result can be: (1) a pure pleasure experience; (2) an experience during which physical or social skills are practiced; (3) an experience in which the child plays with ideas as he explores; and/or (4) an experience involving the weaving of fantasies around objects (toys, persons) in an unconscious attempt to resolve internal conflicts. Play has been likened to dreams.

THERAPIST'S ROLE IN THE PLAY OF THE CHILD

As a therapist, I provide an environment that is designed to foster a state of well-being, with the hope that the child will experience the free flow of energy that is necessary before he can explore his environment with ease. I act as a scientific observer of his play. I note his selection of activities. What is he drawn to? What does he withdraw from? I note his affect (the emotions he experiences as he plays). I listen to the changes in his speech and language, to the quality and intensity of his voice. I ask myself: What stage of development is being reflected in the child's play? What conflicts does he seem to be dealing with? What can I do or say to clarify to both of us what is on the child's mind?

When a drama is being produced, I am ready to play any role assigned to me by the child. As I play the role, I periodically ask questions: "What do I do now? Am I doing it right? Am I crying O.K.?" I, thus, affirm to the child that he is indeed directing the drama and remind him that what is happening is not real. I want to add or subtract as little as possible to or from the child's thoughts, creativity, and affect.

PLAY DISRUPTIONS

Play disruptions signal that the free flow of energy necessary for play has been blocked by internal and/or external forces that are too threatening to the child to allow him to continue that particular play. The disruption may take the form of a simple, but unexpected, change in activity. At other times, the child may suddenly become belligerent or destructive, or demonstrate other kinds of uncontrolled and/or inappropriate behavior. What is happening in the child's play is just too much for him! He is experiencing such a high level of anxiety that impulsiveness reigns and his inner controls can no longer be relied upon. The child is acting out. By definition, acting out is uncontrolled, impulsive behavior that is inappropriate and unacceptable at a particular moment in time and space. The motivating force behind such behavior should be given careful attention by the therapist, but the behavior itself has little significant therapeutic value, and should be stopped. If I sense correctly what caused the disruption, I may be able to reduce the child's anxiety with meaningful words, changing a negative experience to a positive one. If I cannot follow this course, and the child becomes aggressive and/or destructive, I act quickly with words meant to stop this behavior. Those words indicate to him that I do not like his actions, that I have rules and he is breaking them. Storms do not often abate quickly, but it is seldom that I need to restrain a child physically. I am alert to signals that a disruption may occur, and expect the child to respond to my words if it does occur. Once things are back to "normal," I give careful thought to what may have caused the disruption, internally and externally. It often uncovers an important piece of information about the child—and sometimes uncovers an important piece of information about me.

THEMES

Although play is not goal-oriented, it has direction, and as a result of this, themes appear. The following themes may emerge from a child's play: (1) separation-individuation, including the development of object constancy and the fear of losing loved objects; (2) satisfaction of oral needs; (3) control of self, including the control of body functions; (4) fear of damage to body parts; (5) sexual identity and procreation; (6) omnipotence as related to vying for position in the family and in peer groups, and controlling the environment in general; and, (7) coping with rules—developing a conscience. One or many themes may appear in a single therapy session.

SYMBOLIC REPRESENTATIONS

Play themes are sometimes readily apparent. Others may be disguised in the child's effort to protect himself as he plays out thoughts and feelings that may be threatening or painful to him. At these times, he will play, using symbolic representations to screen his thoughts from himself, just as he would do in a dream. Decoding these messages which the child sends to himself is one of my tasks. Breaking the code requires an awareness of what is believed to be the symbolic meaning of objects and actions. If I cannot decode the child's play, viewing his play will be like viewing a foreign movie with no subtitles. What is obvious, I will see. Deeper meanings, I will miss. If I miss the deeper meanings, I miss the opportunity to help the child translate his activities into significant words. These words may be words that the child needs to hear and use if an experience or thought is to be caught and filed away accurately in his memory, ready for future use. An example follows:

Clifford, 9 years, 4 months, chose to play with clay. He created an animal. It had a goat's head, a hippopotamus' body, and a cat's tail. Symbolically, animals are thought to represent some form of impulsiveness. Clifford and I both needed to know more about his animal.

"What do you think of when you think of a goat?' I asked.

"You never know what a goat is going to do next," he said. (I thought: Sounds like mother, but it could be Clifford.)

"What about the hippopotamus?" I asked.

"It's just big. Everybody can see it coming, and better get out of its way."

Clifford had been in treatment, because of stuttering, for one year and 9 months. I knew Clifford and his mother very well. As I thought about the hippopotamus part of Clifford's animal, it seemed to me, again, that it could represent either mother or son. Mom looked very big and powerful to Clifford and Clifford's stuttering behavior loomed large to Mom.

"What about the cat's tail? Let's see . . . when a cat wags his tail . . . what does it mean? Is he happy or sad?" I asked.

"I get mixed up about that. I'm not sure," he said.

I silently recalled that Mom wears a fixed smile on her face whether she is angry or happy. Clifford tends to be a poker-face—unless he is clowning.

I said, "Let's think about this animal of yours. You would have a hard time knowing what he was going to do next, and that would be bad news. He's big enough so that you can see him coming and can deal with him if only to get out of his way. That's sort of good news. You aren't sure whether—when he wags his tail—he is mad or happy, so it would be hard to know how to please him."

"Oh, I remember now! A cat is mad when he wags his tail," he said.

"Do you know anybody who behaves like your animal?" I asked.

"No," he said. He carefully put his animal in his locker and moved to another activity.

My words were first made into questions, in order that Clifford could put significant thoughts about his animal into words. Later my words summarized what he had told me and formed statements as to how I thought some people might feel when coming face to face with this animal. His words, "I remember now! A cat is mad when he wags his tail," spoken fluently, showed some relief in being able to distinguish mad from other feelings. My eagerness to find out who this animal represented put the issue on ice. Clifford's "no" and his careful placement of the now-valued object in his locker, in effect, marked a quiet play disruption. He could not tolerate further exploration of his animal at that moment. Had I waited a little longer for Clifford to say or do something, or had I formed a different question with my words that might have been less threatening, a meaningful piece of play might have continued.

In this example, my awareness of the meaning of symbolic representation first resulted in an expansion of Clifford's play. My words channelled the free, non-goal-oriented flow of energy necessary for play without blocking that flow. This same awareness of the symbolic meaning of play led to a play disruption. A red flag went up when my words suggested an attachment of the play to reality. The free flow of energy was blocked by anxiety. Play was disrupted. This need not be judged as bad or good. It simply reflects the intensity of Clifford's feelings, underlying his play. I do not fear disruptions. Neither do I provoke them. Understood, a disruption can lead to the experiencing of useful insights for both the therapist and the child.

TWO CLINICAL STUDIES

Mary.

Mary was 4 years, 6 months of age when she entered therapy. Her nursery school teachers had difficulty understanding her at times, as did her Daddy. Relationships with peers were poor. They said she "talks funny." She made common substitution errors: j/l, w/r, ə/ɚ, d/ð, f/θ. The sound *l* was sometimes omitted. Vowels were sometimes used incorrectly. She had a pronounced, visible central lisp. Intelligibility was further impaired by a breaking up of some one-syllable words into two syllables. Example: when explaining behavior of a bad mother during an early piece of dramatic play, she said, "θi wʌθ nɑt ə bæjəd mʌdə. θi wʌθ dʒʌjɛθt ɪn ə bæjəd muəd." (She was not a bad mother. She was just in a bad mood.) Language structure and vocabulary were well above the norm.

Expressive speech was blocked at times by repeated "um-ah, um-ah, um-ahs." Occasionally, whole words were repeated. The parents stated that there were times when Mary could not get beyond her "um-ahs" and gave up saying what was on her mind. Mary was seen in therapy twice a week (30-minute sessions) for a total of 77 times. At the end of this period, she entered kindergarten and transferred into a public school speech-language program. At that time, the lisp did not draw attention to itself and the *r* sound was correctly made in some positions. She made no other speech errors. Her speech was fluent.

One theme dominates the following clinical material, which spans 20 therapy sessions. During this interval, one session blended into the next as though there had been no interruption—an obvious sign of the intensity of Mary's interest in the prevailing theme: object constancy.*

The drama began when Mary discovered a little beanbag owl, with a prominent, hooked beak. She held it in her lap as she snacked on a cracker. She said, "This is

---

*Object constancy is a concept that grew out of Piaget's concept of object permanence. It is hypothesized that a very young child views his prime caretaker (designated here as mother) as two objects rather than one. One satisfies his needs and is trustworthy; the other is a source of distress and is not to be trusted. The child sees the former as "good," the latter as "bad." When he views his mother as "bad," he loses his "good" mother; when he views his mother as "good," his "bad" mother disappears. With time, the child who develops normally emotionally, finds that his "good" mother and his "bad" mother are indeed the same person and he need not reject or lose one or the other. Essentially, then, when a specific, vital human object remains constant to the child, regardless of impulsive feelings he experiences about that object, object constancy is achieved. It is further hypothesized that when the child achieves object constancy in regard to his prime caretaker, he can better accept the bad and good within important "others," including himself.

a baby and I'm going to feed it." She put a cracker to its mouth. Suddenly, she took the cracker out of the baby's mouth and tried to stuff a paper wrapper in its mouth instead. She then pushed the baby into my hands, and said I was to make sounds for the baby. I was to cry and scream because I did not like paper. Then, she said, I would be the good mother and the baby would be the bad baby and she would be the bad mother.

The next session, Mary brought a stuffed animal from home. The new baby, a girl, was a good baby. Every session thereafter, Mary brought a different stuffed animal, who was the good baby. The bad baby always remained the same. Mary said it was neither a boy nor a girl, but I was to call it "him." At the end of each session, he was carefully put away in Mary's locker.

The bad mother was very sweet to the good baby. The good baby was very polite and did everything the bad mother told her to do. She only cried when the bad baby woke her up with his loud screams. The bad baby was to do many bad things. Mary's script dictated that the baby was very proud of his "nose." The bad mother became her angriest when he joyously sang, "I love my nose! I love my nose!" For this behavior, for shouting bad words, for just crying and screaming, the bad mother continually threatened the bad baby. She said she would put him in jail—send him into outer space—poison him—send him to the disposal room—put him in the garbage can. The biggest insult of all was to tell the bad baby he was nothing but a bean bag! As the good mother, I could not comfort or protect my bad baby. I could say I loved him, but I could not fondle him. I was to be continually angry with the baby because he was continually bad.

Then came the final scene of this many-act drama. My bad baby was keeping the good baby from sleeping. I was to shake my baby and shout insults and threats to him. At the same time, Mary held her good baby tenderly and sang "Love-a-bye and Goodnight." Mary had created a musical score, a counterpoint, uniting good and bad. Both love and anger could survive in harmony without losing the power each possessed.

Throughout Mary's 8 months of therapy, her words and my words labeled her amorphous thoughts and feelings. In the process, Mary's articulation improved and fluency was attained. Goals I had set for Mary and myself had been achieved.

Sarah.

Sarah came into treatment at 5 years of age because of a very severe speech and language disorder. Only her mother could understand her—some of the time. She entered kindergarten with the expectation that she might have to be transferred into a special classroom. At this writing, she is 7 and 1/2 years old, repeating first grade in the regular classroom. A recent report card showed: reading, excellent; spelling, excellent; language skills, satisfactory; mathematics, outstanding. The teacher's chief complaint is that Sarah talks too much. The session that follows took place when Sarah was 7 years old.

Sarah pushed the door open and came bursting into the therapy room. Wearing a broad grin, with her beautiful, freckled face upturned, her blue eyes sparkling, and a little breathless from running as fast as she was able, she shouted, "I saw you! I saw you! I saw you when I was in my car. Didn't you hear me pounding on my window! You were talking to a *man*!" What she had viewed was a brief, but animated conversation between two friends. Sarah had never before seen me talk to a man, other than her father, and had rarely seen me outside the office.

Sarah settled down and turned her attention to the toy cupboard where she picked up and examined a barn. Discovering that one of the barn doors no longer swung open without falling out of position, she said "Look! This is broken! Get me some Scotch tape." She worked silently, her tongue actively moving as she concentrated on her task. Her first efforts were failures. She scowled and pressed her lips together and gave a stifled sigh, *but* she persevered. As I watched, it seemed to me that her present course was bound to meet with more failures. "I think I see something you can do. Can I help?" I asked. "No! Be quiet! Don't talk!" she shouted. She continued her repair work as I quietly watched. At last, success! I clapped my hands. Sarah smiled, but chastisingly said, "Not yet!"

She added one more piece of tape and proudly patted it into place. She checked out her work to make sure she had done the job. I said, "That's really good, Sarah! That barn door was damaged and you repaired it!" She looked pleased, picked up the barn, and replaced it in the toy cupboard.

A piece of tape had stuck to the back of her sunsuit—an outfit that she had once proudly told me was just like her mother's. The top was strapless, drawing attention to the bust line. A look of concern crossed her face as her hand searched for the tape she could not see. Once she found it, she whined and winced as she peeled it off, rolled it up, and threw it into the waste basket. She whirled around, facing me. With her arms close to her body and a look of distress on her face, she set all her body parts in motion. She quickly pulled down the top of her suit, glanced at herself and me, and then quickly brought the top back into position. She ran toward the couch and threw herself onto it, kicked her feet and made noises bordering on crying sounds.

"What's happened?" I asked. "I told you about the tape. You pulled it off and threw it away, did a kind of a dance, pulled your top down and up and now you're lying on the couch as though you were sad . . . or maybe mad."

"I don't feel good!" she whined.

She hugged a pillow and curled up into a ball.

"Tell me about that," I said.

"I just don't feel good!" she said, with less of a whine in her voice.

"Maybe you feel damaged, too, and in need of repair. Can I do something to help?"

She did not respond verbally, but began to rearrange the pillows to make the couch more comfortable.

"I see you want to take care of yourself. You're going to start by making yourself more comfortable," I said.

After lying still for a few minutes, she sat up, stood up and patted the pillows in place, and then slowly, with shoulders slightly drooped, eyes down, she walked toward the game cupboard. She opened the door and took out the board games one by one. She looked inside the first one, rejected it, and threw it out toward me, somewhat defiantly.

"I can see that you don't want to play with *that* one!" I said. My words not only acknowledged Sarah's outburst of anger, but also reminded her of the task she had set for herself—that of finding a game that would relieve her discomfort.

"I see one board you won't have to open because it has a label on it," I said. "And now you can read!"

She immediately chose this game to play. Before the game began, she announced, "You can't move in front of me!"

"That's your rule for this game? O.K. You're the boss of the game! I'll follow your rules," I said.

The game involved taking chips out of a grab bag. As she took her first turn, she pouted, half-scowling, looking off in one direction and then seemingly returning her attention reluctantly to what she was doing. I said, "You look mad, Sarah."

"I don't know which one I'm going to get," she said angrily, and almost painfully.

"Oh!" I said, "You're not mad. You're wondering if you should peek or not."

Sarah laughed and said, "I'm not peeking!" and continued the game.

Sarah's emotions were now on an even keel. She was willing to follow an established rule of the game and I followed the rule she had laid down for me. If I had the opportunity to move ahead, I lost my turn. I said "Sometimes it feels good to know you can make the rules. You can control what happens." She showed great interest in reading all the printed matter on the board. When time was up, she left easily, greeting her mother and brother warmly.

Several themes appear in this therapy session: sexual identity, fear of damage to the body, and control of the environment. The session actually began with Sarah's observation of me, outside my office building, talking to a friend. Her excited behavior could have been the result of seeing me as a part of her outside world, and/or seeing me as a woman talking to a man. The intensity of her drive to get to me as quickly as possible could have begun with the frustration of her audible and visible efforts to get my attention without success. Separations have been difficult for Sarah. Anticipating a connection she was sure she was going to make ("I saw you!") excited and pleased her.

Her play led her to the repairing of a damaged part of a barn. The action that followed her awareness that tape used to repair the barn was stuck on her clothing could be interpreted symbolically to reflect her fear of possible damage to herself. The brief exposure of her "breasts" indicated an awareness that, one day, she would look like her Mommy. She must have been disappointed when she could see that, so far, she looked no different from her two brothers.

She took to the couch, saying she felt bad, and found comfort in loving the pillows and moving into the fetal position. Her behavior showed relief when I suggested that she might feel damaged and in need of repair. She knew I was standing by to help and was also reminded indirectly that she had repaired damage to the barn earlier and, perhaps, could tend to her own needs as well.

She moved to a game over which she knew, from past experience, she could have control. Anxiety lessened. Her rules guaranteed that she would not suffer a loss. She could now draw her attention to a 7-year-old task—mastery of an academic skill—by pouring her energy into reading the messages written on the game board. At the end of the session, she stepped out, ready to cope with her outside world.

The free flow of energy Sarah brought with her to the session carried her into troubled areas. I knew Sarah very well, having watched, listened, and interacted with her for two years. My knowledge that symbolic meaning can be attached to spontaneous behavior made it possible for me to verbalize enough to help her cope with what appeared, at first, to be intolerable to her. My verbalizations, in most cases, were nothing more than verbal pictures of what I saw happening, including the affect Sarah seemed to be experiencing as she played. Sarah's words and my words brought each "picture" into focus. Sarah's therapeutic experiences were now labeled and could be effectively, accurately, and selectively stored in Sarah's memory, ready for future use, should the need arise. My words were well-articulated, spontaneously and creatively structured, thoughtfully chosen words. Sarah's words were an integral part of her. Her improved speech and language reflected the fact that she had heard my normal speech and was identifying with me and my normal speech patterns.

No claim is made that the use of the therapy I have described will bring about normal speech and language for all children with communication disorders. Dramatic changes can take place, however. I have found that the method affords unusual opportunities to make use of words that are uniquely important to each patient. Vocabulary, therefore, is built upon the needs of the child. As he effectively uses this vocabulary, a new world opens up for him and his family. He puts order into his world through meaningful words, and with order can come improved language, articulation, voice, and fluency.

SELECTED REFERENCES

Cohen, D., and Stern, S. *Oberving and Recording the Behavior of Young Children.* New York; Teachers College Press, 1978.

Cooper, S., and Wanerman, L. *Children in Treatment.* New York; Brunner/Mazel, 1977.

Garvey, C. *Play.* Cambridge, Massachusetts: Harvard University Press, 1977.

Greenspan, S., and Greenspan, N. *The Clinical Interview of the Child.* New York: McGraw-Hill Book Company, 1981.

Kaplan, L., *Oneness and Separateness: From Infant to Individual.* New York: Simon and Schuster, 1978.

CHAPTER EIGHT

EVALUATION OF THERAPEUTIC OUTCOME

Method of Gerald M. Siegel

THERAPEUTIC OUTCOME

The measurement of therapeutic outcome can be approached in two rather different ways. In one, outcome is evaluated against a specific target: stutter-free speech, normal pitch, correct articulation. This approach deals in absolutes that are unattainable by many clients. The second approach is not as neat, but is more reasonable. It defines outcome in relative terms and focuses more on the course of improvement than on a terminal goal. I prefer the second approach because it is more compatible with the view of therapy as a process.

For many clients, communication difficulties will persist throughout their lives. Outcome is an ambiguous construct when applied to aphasia, severe hearing loss, mental retardation, and other severe communication disorders. Improvement for almost any communication disorder typically proceeds irregularly, in spurts, plateaus, and even reversals. Progress should be defined by the slope rather than the client's place on the curve. A plateau following slow, labored improvement may mean that progress has ground to a halt and new methods are needed. A plateau following a period of accelerated improvement may signify that the client is consolidating new skills. Considerations like these require that assessment be designed as an integral and continuing part of therapy, and not merely as a measure of outcome.

COMMUNICATION DISORDERS

Communication disorders is a cross-roads discipline that stands at the intersection of many applied and basic fields. As a consequence, we are affected by current research and theory in other professions. For example, theories of language have gone through several intellectual upheavals in the last half century, and this is reflected in methods of language assessment. Earlier, we evaluated language by the count and tally methods that dominated child development, and focused on vocabulary size, length of utterance, and inventories of words, sentences, and speech sounds. The linguist Chomsky's influence in the late 1950s led to measurement techniques that emphasized the rule-governed nature of language, and particularly syntax. More recently, the urgent themes in psycholinguistics have been semantics and pragmatics, and these have influenced measurement approaches in language disorders.

The fact that we are amenable to changes in other fields is both frustrating and exhilarating. Our technology seems never to be in place. We no sooner mastered the intricacies of behavioral methodology when we were invaded by psycholinguistics. Tests of syntax were barely off the presses when the pragmatics campaign began. To the extent that new ideas in communication and language theory have any practical implications at all, they find their way into our journals and our clinical procedures. Increasingly, the basic disciplines look toward applied fields for confirmation of theoretical principles, and so we have become the testing ground for many new concepts and approaches that are developed elsewhere.

Of course, not everything that appears under a new label is actually new; nor is everything that is old necessarily to be discarded. The field of communication disorders has always emphasized the communicative functions of speech, hearing, and language. The danger was that we might set aside our traditional concern for communication and become swept up in formal, structural approaches. The pragmatics that is generating so much enthusiasm in psycholinguistics is nothing less than the bedrock of the field of communication disorders, and has always been so. Measurement in our field is anchored in the communicative aspects of language. Assessment methods do not long survive if they do not lead to insights or techniques that are relevant for communication adequacy.

INTERPERSONAL COMMUNICATION

Communication, by definition, involves both a transmitter and a receiver of information. Furthermore, speaking and listening are constantly in flux during normal conversation. To complicate affairs further, speakers are usually simultaneously listeners with respect to their own communication attempts. Formal assessment methods typically try to reduce this complexity through test formats that fix attention on either the speaking or hearing roles. Thus, articulation tests are usually administered in quiet environments. The child being tested is required to listen very carefully, and only then to respond. Distractions are kept to a minimum and optimal performance is sought. Outside of the clinic, however, the same child will be speaking in a noisy environment, competing with others for attention, and formulating, as well as uttering, speech.

The speech that occurs in normal conversation may be too unpredictable and chaotic for comprehensive analysis. Not all of the sounds or words that need to be measured will appear on the playground or in the lunchroom. Some linguistic forms are improbable in natural speech. Variations in pitch and loudness are constrained by the situation in which the child is talking. In order to determine the limits of a child's performance, it will also be necessary to devise formal, structured test situations. We know, however, that context and situation influence performance, and it is important to incorporate this knowledge into assessment approaches.

RANGE OF PERFORMANCE

Features of the environment can be included in the testing method. For example, some tests of speech sound production require the child to say the test words in quiet and in a noisy background. Response in noise provides a good prediction of how stable a newly acquired articulation skill has become. If speech breaks down under noise in a test situation, it is likely to break down over a summer vacation without therapy. Similar modifications can be made in test formats for other communication disorders. The point is not to devise a context that will force a breakdown in performance, but to sample the behavior in a variety of contexts.

It is important to have a feeling for the best performance the client can produce in ideal test situations, and also to evaluate performance in ordinary and in demanding environments. Both ends of the continuum are significant. Children's syntax in an imitation task is significantly improved when the children are allowed to look at relevant pictures before imitating the examiner's test utterances. Using pictures or some other context in this way gives a more accurate picture of what the child is capable of doing. It is useful to have this information, as well as how he ordinarily performs. We can use context systematically, then, to evaluate the child's performance in situations that range from optimal to difficult. This will provide information about both the range and the stability of the client's abilities.

LISTENER RESPONSE

The fact that speech is basically an interpersonal behavior suggests another assessment method that should be appropriate for a variety of disorders. It is possible to set up situations in which speech is measured explicitly in terms of its effect on a listener. Most language assessment methods carefully inventory the client's responses to specific items. We tally and describe disfluencies, record the frequency of correct and incorrect articulations, describe voice and quality characteristics, etc. These attributes are important, presumably, because they affect the listener, but it is rare to bring the listener into the evaluation process, except for the trained ears of the clinician.

Communication research has developed a measure of referential communication that has interesting possibilities for the clinician. The basic paradigm involves a speaker and a listener who are required to solve a problem based on the information transmitted by the speaker. Perhaps they are both supposed to arrange items on a board in exactly the same sequence, or must select the same ambiguous drawing from a cluster of similar drawings, or identify a face or picture that is being described. In this task, communication adequacy is defined in terms of the listener's performance. A measure of the client's severity at the outset of therapy might be how well he communicates in such tasks, and improvement can be stated in terms of increasing accuracy in generating correct listener responses. It is sometimes difficult to specify the gains a client has made over the course of therapy. Clients may learn subtle ways to improve communication that elude formal descriptive measures, but do have an impact on listeners. The interpersonal paradigm could reveal such changes.

GENERALIZATION

Context also comes up in considerations of generalization. How can we determine whether the gains the client is displaying in the clinic are generalizing to the larger social world? Increasing attention is being devoted to methods to promote and assess generalization. The problems are legion. The clinician cannot follow the client into every social situation. Hidden recording devices may have some value, but they also constitute a potential invasion of privacy. Furthermore, they are cumbersome and a bother. Parental or client report is a source of information, but is subject to obvious sources of bias. It would seem that some form of frequent and perhaps covert monitoring of the client's behavior is necessary to obtain an accurate indication of his communication behavior outside the clinic. At the very least, the client should be returned to the clinic for frequent evaluations, spread over a long period of time. Communication disorders like stuttering are notorious for their episodic nature. This surely helps to account for the perplexing finding that many more stutterers are successfully treated than remain cured. Indeed, in some instances the same stutterer can account for several successful cures, as he goes from one therapy program to another, in search of the ultimate cure.

In addition to frequent monitoring over an extended period, it is possible to build tests of generalization into the formal assessment methods used in the clinic. The client can be asked to speak in front of an audience, to imagine a difficult or stressful situation, to talk in the presence of noise or frequent interruptions, and so on. Although these devices do not mimic the experiences that will be encountered outside the clinic, they can provide an approximation to the stresses of real-world communication. In addition, they may be useful therapeutic devices.

BEHAVIOR VERSUS ATTITUDES

The behavioristic approach that characterized social sciences for so many years left its mark on communication disorders as well. Subjective statements about feelings, emotions, and attitudes were largely eschewed in favor of empirical descriptions of observable behavior. Clinicians scrupulously avoided talking with stutterers about anxieties or speech-related fears lest this contaminate purely behavioral treatment methods. Attitude scales were taboo. When attitudes were acknowledged as existing, they were invariably placed within quotations, and were considered epiphenomena, secondary to the observable responses. Or they were treated as verbal behaviors and subject to laws of verbal conditioning. Thus, to eliminate "fear of speaking," punish all verbal responses that allude to "fear." Or, more conveniently, references to fear can be diminished by reducing the stuttering that precipitates the references. But the attitudes themselves were not acceptable in the clinical domain—except that most clinicians could not deny their clients the honest expression of feelings, and so, in various guises, attitudes crept back into the clinical enterprise.

Attitude should be acknowledged as a formal partner in therapy. A client's statements about himself and his perception of his progress in therapy are important elements that deserve consideration in therapy. For one thing, they are significant prognosticators. Clients who feel that they are doing well and express confidence that they can improve are likely to show gains, more than those who are pessimistic and skeptical. On the other hand, if the client consistently gives glowing reports of his improvement, none of which is evident in his behavior, that might suggest that he does not have the same attitudes and goals as the clinician, and it may be necessary to come to some common agreement about the purpose of therapy. This is not to say that the clinician's attitudes must prevail. But if clinician and client are on a different course, this should certainly be recognized. In the same way, I think it is valuable to know the attitudes of significant people in the client's environment. If a husband thinks a husky voice is charming in his wife, then the clinician's efforts may be futile. If parents think that silence is golden in a young cleft palate child, then speaking assignments may have little chance of success. I have worked diligently with a misarticulating child, only to discover that her mother considered a nondistorted /s/ to sound unnatural in her daughter.

Speech is not an insulated activity. It serves a complex social purpose. The feelings the client has about himself as a speaker and about his accomplishments in therapy are important data for a client and the clinician to consider in coming to some evaluation of therapy. A fluent speaker who does not feel he is fluent has a problem.

DESIGN OF ASSESSMENT PROCEDURES

There are many approaches to designing an assessment strategy, and they are not always compatible. Clinicians need not invariably proceed from the same framework, but it may be useful to review some of the reasons for assessment. Perhaps the most compelling is to identify communication problems in a way that will influence the design of a therapy program. Standard scores, percentiles, and normative comparisons are of limited value if they do not highlight the communication deficiencies that need to be remediated. I find little value in a test that indicates a child is very deviant, but provides no clues concerning the components that lead to that deviancy and does not point the way to therapy. We have for too long been constrained by the need to describe communication adequacy in terms of standardized, normed, formal assessment devices that yield up a score. It is much more important to provide a profile. More often than not we know that a child is significantly retarded in communication skills, but we do not know what features of communication are deficient. This is more important than a norm-based general score.

If assessment is to be useful in evaluation of language, for example, it must proceed from some model of communication. Not all clinicians will agree about the particulars of such a model, but some variant is necessary so that the clinician can be guided in an approach to assessment. Basically, the model incorporates the features of communication that the clinician has come to regard as important for successful performance. These may involve phonology, morphology, syntax, semantics, and pragmatics. Or, it may include specific subsets of these. Or, it may focus on preverbal skills that are thought to be prerequisites of communication. We seem to be far from a theory of communication that can comprehensively guide us in assessment and therapy, but a model is surely within reach. Clinicians who unthinkingly use a particular test or battery of tests for every client will, unknowingly, have allowed their conception of language to be guided entirely by the dimensions of the battery. Far better to develop such a model and then use tests selectively as needed to fill out the dimensions of the model.

In designing an assessment approach for a given client, the clinician should keep all options open. Commercial tests are time-savers and a great comfort as well. But they rarely tell all that is needed about a client's performance. The clinician has to be agile, jumping from procedure to procedure, using what is useful and discarding what is not, without being intimidated by the formal aspects of test development. It is important to understand the meaning of standardization and the development of norms for a test, but not to be enslaved by them. When normative data are required, the clinician should be able to administer a test precisely as it is described. But she should also be able to use tests creatively to serve the assessment needs of a particular client. This will almost invariably also mean going beyond the realm of commercial instruments. It is seldom that a test will probe precisely the behavior of interest in sufficient depth to be used exclusively. Clinicians must devise their own assessment methods, with full consideration of their limitations, but with the confidence that they can put clinical intuitions and insights to work in devising methods that are informative and linked to intervention methods.

SELECTED REFERENCES

Darley, F., Fay, W., Newman, P., Rees, M., and Siegel, G. *Evaluation of Appraisal Techniques in Speech and Language Pathology*. Reading, Mass.: Addison-Wesley, 1979.

Miller, J. *Assessing Language Production in Children*. Baltimore: University Park Press, 1981.

Siegel, G., and Broen, P. Language Assessment. In L. Lloyd (Ed.), *Communication and Assessment Strategies*. Baltimore: University Park Press, 1976.

INDEX